JimsHealthAndMuscle.com

Barbell

&

Dumbbell Training

A Weight Training Guide For Strength & Fitness That Won't Go Out Of Fashion.

James Atkinson

CONTENTS

Section 1

Why Barbells and dumbbells?

Among the many benefits of barbell and dumbbell training, here are a few of the big ones:

- Increased strength.
- Increased mobility.
- Correction of poor posture.
- Development in balance and dexterity.
- Increased muscle mass.
- Change of body composition (less fat, more lean muscle).
- The protection of joints.
- Increased self-confidence.

What will you learn?

- Why choose barbells and dumbbells
- How to train correctly with barbells and dumbbells
- How to train efficiently for your unique fitness goals
- How to create and plan your own training routine using dumbbells and barbells
- How to avoid training plateaus for continued development
- How to perform each exercise correctly to avoid injury and maximise results

Other essential elements, such as:

- Full body workouts
- Split routines
- Drop sets, supersets and giant sets
- Core strength and abdominal development

Barbells and dumbbells are an excellent choice for any weight trainer. There are many benefits to training with free weights that you will get for muscular development when compared to other training equipment, like resistance bands or even bodyweight.

Muscular development is a term that's often miss interpreted. I speak from experience when I say that this term, when mentioned in conjunction with barbell or dumbbell training, can often cause new trainers in particular to immediately resist or show some reluctance to entertain this type of exercise.

As a personal trainer, I have experienced a fair few clients tell me they "don't want to look like Arnold" so they don't want to train with dumbbells or barbells. This is probably down to their interpretation of the term "muscular development".

So what is muscular development, really? The term is not exclusive to bodybuilder physiques. It means increased:

- Muscle strength
- Muscle tone
- Muscle growth
- Muscle flexibility
- Skeletal and joint support
- Overall muscle function

When you look at the above list, I'm sure you would agree that everyone, bodybuilder or not, would like to feel the benefits of every point there.

When used correctly, barbells and dumbbells are the number one choice for weight training, and I'm sure that as long as humanity is interested in fitness and any aspect of muscular development, this type of exercise will remain the bread and butter of the health and fitness industry… And I hope, references to "Arnold" in this setting will stick around too!

So why are barbells and dumbbells the number one choice for weight training and muscle development? The simple answer is that the heavier you can lift, the stronger your muscles will become. This does not mean that you lift so heavy at every opportunity that you damage yourself. There is a balance and the resistance level will change from person to person and ability to ability. This will be explained later.

The fact is that the designed nature of barbells and dumbbells gives us the opportunity to lift at a resistance level that is very well suited to gains in muscle development. The movements and exercises that we can perform with these free weights lets us maximise our training effect.

Barbells

Barbells range in length, thickness and weight. There are barbells that have a fixed weight. These normally come in a set, barbells that are half and three quarter length, and barbells that are not exactly straight, like the EZ bar.

The standard and most versatile is the Olympic bar. It weighs 20 kg, has a length of about 7 feet and a grip thickness is around 1 inch. It's a fairly chunky piece of kit when compared to some of the other common options.

We will look at a few other types of specialist barbell such as the EZ barbell, but the primary focus of illustrations and exercise description will be on the Olympic bar, although every barbell exercise that's mentioned can be performed with any type of straight barbell.

Barbell exercises are great for big compound movements to increase strength. The solid, straight bar allows us to load up bigger weights and although stabiliser muscles are used, there is not as much focus on them in these lifts as the same lifts when performed with dumbbells.

For the beginner, barbells are a great way to develop exercise form with compound movements, but there are drawbacks. We will get into this in a later chapter.

Dumbbells

Dumbbells also come in different shapes and sizes. These days, the most common ones in gyms are the fixed weight type, and they are definitely the most convenient and easy to use. These are not practical for most people who want to stick to home workouts with dumbbells, as a lot of space is needed.

For home workouts and home gyms with limited space, it's probably best to invest in the plate loaded kind. These are basically short, one handed barbells that usually weigh about 2.5 kgs and have small weighted discs ready to be loaded on.

Dumbbell exercises give us the opportunity to increase range of movement, focus on single muscle exercises and offer more development of our stabiliser muscles. As they are independent weights, we can target single limbs to even out any weaknesses. So when a training routine is set up using both barbells and dumbbells, we really have a great opportunity to optimise our training progression.

Health Check

Before you embark on any fitness routine, please consult your Doctor or physiotherapist. If you have any health conditions, always check if the type of exercise and exercise choices you intend to involve yourself with.

1. Do not exercise if you are unwell.

2. Stop if you feel pain, and if the pain does not subside, consult your doctor or physiotherapist.

3. Do not exercise if you have taken alcohol or had a large meal in the last few hours.

4. If you are taking medication, please check with your doctor to make sure it is okay for you to exercise.

5. If in doubt at all, please check with your Doctor or physiotherapist first – you may even want to take this routine and go through it with them. It may be helpful to ask for a blood pressure, cholesterol and weight check. You can then have these taken again in a few months to see the benefit.

Barbells Or Dumbbells?

When introduced to barbell training for the first time, some trainers may find certain exercises slightly uncomfortable. I have personal experience of this, and it was never explained to me. It was only through extended time training with barbells and my experience training others that it finally made sense.

We are not all made the same. Some of us are taller, some shorter, some have longer limbs up top than down bottom and some of us even have specific conditions affecting our natural movement. With this in mind, training with barbells can be more difficult for some people than for others.

The potential problem with barbell training is that the movement of an exercise can force our joints into an unnatural position. This can be a big problem in some circumstances, but it can be a good thing in others. Let's look at shoulder press as an example, the potential problems and potential benefits:

To perform a shoulder press, we start with the bar at chin level with a grip space just wider than our shoulders.

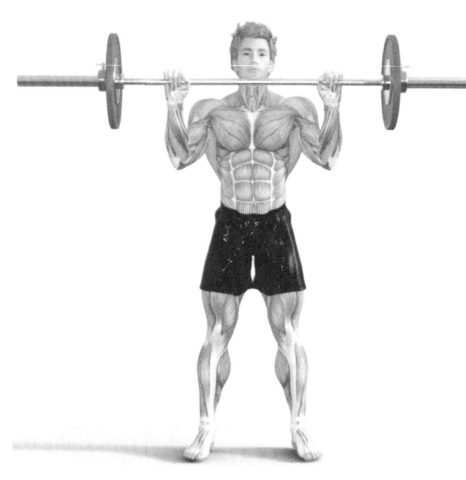

We then push the bar above our head to engage our shoulder muscles.

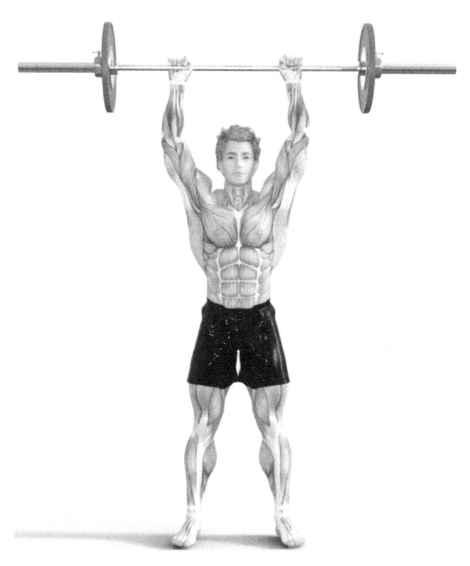

As you can see, our wrists are forced into a position that's dictated by the solid bar. This is where there can be potential problems for some. If the trainer has limited movement in the rotation of their wrist, it can have a knock on effect through the entire arm into the shoulder. This not only causes discomfort for the trainer, but can change the form of the exercise, diluting the effect to the shoulders, cause injury or if this is done for any length of time, train the body to develop an imbalance of muscular strength. Developing stronger front deltoids and neglecting the rear is a good example of what can happen with muscular imbalance.

The same issue of forcing our joints into a fixed position when using a barbell for some exercises can actually be a tremendous benefit for other trainers. This is from a posture, mobility and flexibility point of view. If the trainer has no "mechanical" issues but finds it uncomfortable to perform an exercise with a barbell, they should consider the flexibility and mobility of their joints.

Let's stick with the barbell shoulder press to highlight this potential benefit. If the trainer has rounded shoulders because of poor posture bought on by any number of things, or has weak rear deltoids through under use, or even tight forearm flexors and extensors that limits wrist rotation, training with a barbell and performing regular shoulder press, could help to fix these problems.

There is a well-known phrase that I always fall back to with muscle development and that is: "Use it or lose it"

If you don't use a muscle, it will atrophy (shrink and weaken). Muscles that are not regularly challenged will not function as they should, so they will not support the skeleton optimally. Going back to the shoulder press exercise, in everyday life, for many people, lifting objects directly above their head is not commonplace, and the shoulder press movement, when performed correctly engages all three heads of the shoulder muscle, front, middle and rear.

Lifting our arms out in front of us is a far more common occurrence and this engages the front shoulder muscle. This means that most people have stronger front shoulder muscles than rear, which can cause rounding of the shoulders.

Stronger front shoulder muscles mean you are far more likely to subconsciously use these for activities and everyday tasks, which further increases the issue.

On top of this, if we are not aware of our flexibility and do not use our body to its full potential, we will risk losing flexibility. So for this situation, the restrictive nature of barbell exercises can actually help us increase mobility, engage and strengthen muscles that are being neglected, and help correct poor posture to give us a whole bunch of benefits to our fitness levels.

We can do the same exercise with dumbbells, but as it is with a barbell, there are potential issues and potential benefits. Let's look at the exercise before we get into these.

Below is the start position. As you can see, it's very similar to the barbell position:

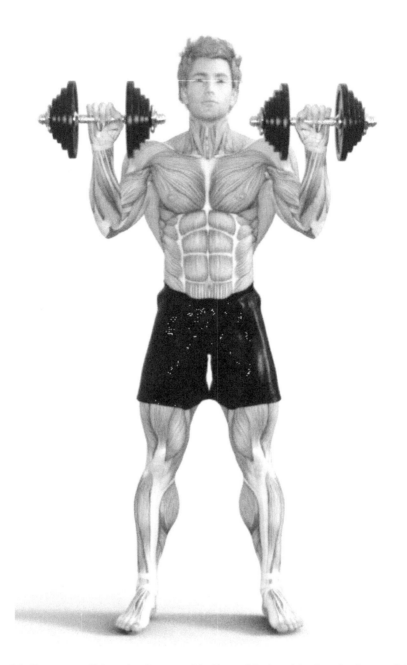

Dumbbells are parallel to the floor and in line with the chin, just in front of the shoulders. Some people may have a starting position where the discs will actually touch the front of the shoulder.

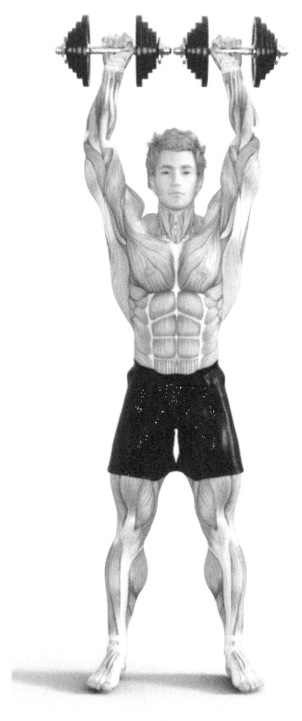

The above picture shows the top of the movement. As you can see, the hands can be moved across the body's midline through the movement, so the inner ends of the dumbbells touch at the top of the movement.

Using dumbbells as opposed to barbells gives us more movement potential, and as they are independent, we will use more stabiliser muscles to perform a movement. With this example, while we push the dumbbells above our head, our wrists need to maintain their position, our shoulders need to work a bit more to stop the weight from pulling them too far backwards or forwards and our elbows need to be stable to stop the weight falling to either side.

So in a nutshell, there is a lot more going on with a dumbbell shoulder press than there is with a barbell shoulder press, and this is true for most dumbbell exercises when compared to barbell exercises.

The extra need for stabilisation when performing dumbbell exercises is largely a benefit with muscle development, but there are more benefits to training with dumbbells that relate to the mechanics of an individual's body.

An example of this is for someone with limited wrist or shoulder rotation. Limited joint rotation can be because of tight or weak muscle groups and can be fixed with the right mobility and strength training. But it can also be because of the ergonomics of an individual's body.

If it's a question of ergonomics, may be much more comfortable for some trainers to do their lifts with dumbbells rather than barbells. With the example of a shoulder press, and adding the example of limited wrist rotation, dumbbells can be far more comfortable to perform than barbell shoulder press. The trainer can still perform a good shoulder press with their wrists turned slightly in to the body as there is no straight bar forcing them to over rotate their wrists.

Below is an example of a shoulder press done with limited wrist movement. Note the dumbbell position.

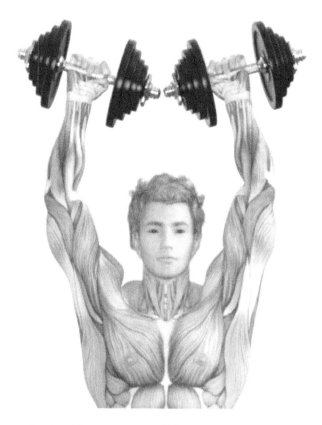

As you can see, the shoulder press can still be performed effectively by someone with limited movement due to joint injury or genetic makeup. For some trainers, this may be a better option for shoulder press than doing the same movement with a barbell.

If there is a limited joint movement due to lack of flexibility or muscle weakness in some trainers, I would suggest that using a barbell could actually be a better choice, as it may work to fix this problem. But this has to be decided on an individual level.

There is an argument that dumbbells are better than barbells, but in my opinion, they both have their benefits, and therefore I would recommend the use of both. Try the different exercises and decide which one is right for you for each muscle group. It's great to have a variety of movements to choose from when planning your workouts.

Whichever option you choose, you should always aim for correct exercise form and range of motion. Always be aware that training with dumbbells can take more concentration and thought as you will work against gravity on several more dimensions than that of a barbell.

Exercise Form, Mechanics & Workload

In every guide that I've written, podcast episode recorded and training article published about exercise, I've been relentless about correct form. I believe that the correct exercise form is the number one priority when engaging in resistance training, especially with free weights.

Incorrect exercise form can be bad for several reasons. The first and most obvious reason is the increased risk of injury. Bad backs and rotator cuff issues are amongst the most common. I've trained in lots of different gyms over the years and have actually, impulsively winced at times watching trainers using bad exercise techniques, whilst often lifting more weight than they can safely handle.

The second and more insidious problem when lifting weights with incorrect form is that it can lead to poor posture, reduce flexibility and other related issues. If you train with a poor exercise form for long enough and avoid injury or pain, your muscles will develop, but they will develop according to your training.

A great example that everyone should be able to relate to about correct form is the simple act of walking. Walking is an activity we all do without thinking about it. Although there are no weights involved, we are still using a bunch of muscle groups. For example, if you're walking style is more focused on bearing weight through your toes, you will work your calves more and your glutes and quads will have an easier time, so will develop less, if your feet pronate (toes face in to your body's midline), you will focus the workload onto your inner quads and weaknesses will develop through the rest of your leg muscles. The longer we are unaware of our condition, the more solidified it will become. Muscles doing the work will strengthen and muscles being neglected will not be challenged, so they have the potential to weaken, shorten or atrophy.

There are many examples of issues with walking, but hopefully this brief and basic overview highlights the potential problems that can be caused and shows that a little thought and knowledge of body mechanics can probably correct bad habits. At this point, I want to acknowledge something that was mentioned earlier, and that is that everyone's made slightly differently. There are cases where an individual's genetics force them into certain positions, so correcting form may not be as simple for some than others; again, this has to be assessed on an individual basis.

The best way to approach weight training and exercise form is to understand that every exercise targets specific muscle groups and that each exercise is related to a movement that the body can perform.

In everyday weight training, every rep of every set should be performed to the best of the body's ability to target the muscle group being worked, whilst working within the target workload and full range of motion.

Here are the elements of a safe and effective exercise movement:

Body positioning

Each exercise has a "start" and a "top of movement" position. When starting a set of any exercise, it's really important to take the time to set yourself up correctly. In this guide, each exercise description has two illustrations showing the start the position and the top of movement position.

Study the guide and make sure you understand which muscle group is going to be targeted and familiarise yourself with the start position and top of movement position.

Big mirrors in gyms are not there for people to check out how big their biceps are, they are there so trainers can check their exercise form, so make good use of them for this, check your start position, perform a few reps with no weights to ensure you are keeping the correct position throughout the movement.

Range of motion

Every muscle in the human body has a maximum extension and maximum contraction, so it's important to work the muscle through this entire range where possible. We want to aim for "full range of motion" when performing resistance exercises.

Here is an example of a full range of motion using barbell curls:

This is the start position: flat back, abs engaged, looking forward and ready to start our set of barbell bicep curls. Biceps are our focus for this exercise, so take a look at the full extension. The arm is fully straightened to where the elbows are about to lock out, so the tension is already on the bicep.

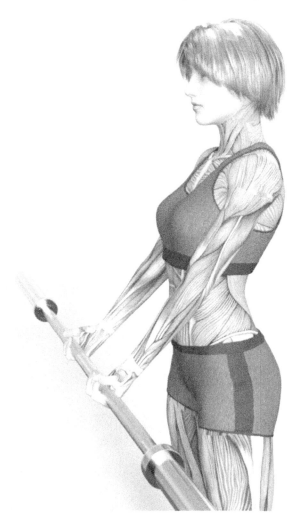

At the top of the movement, we are looking for maximum contraction. This is the point when you have a good squeeze on the bicep. The range of movement with bicep curls should normally be just before the forearms are at right angles to the floor, but depending on the person, it could continue to just past this. One thing to note on exercises like this is that we are working against gravity to stimulate the muscle, so if you go beyond the right angle point, the tension may be lost slightly.

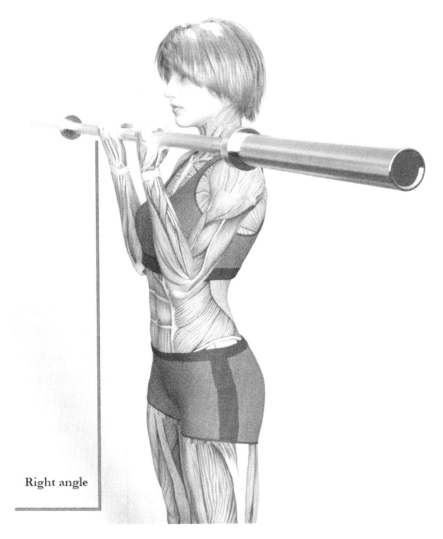

Right angle

"Cheat reps", "baby reps", "21s" and "pulsing" are all exercise methods used to try to stimulate the muscle further once it is fatigued. But to be honest, I believe there are far more effective ways to do this whilst maintaining a full range of movement exercises. We will look at how to get the most out of the full range of movement methods later.

Target workload

Working within your target workload is another vital element of muscular development that needs to be considered. The most basic way to put this is – If you are not lifting heavy enough, your muscles won't develop. If you are lifting too heavy, you lose form and range of motion so are not getting the benefits you could be. There is a sweet spot for everyone on every exercise.

It's true to say that the heavier the weights you are training with, the stronger and more developed you will become. But you need to consider all the other elements in this section too. You need to lift with correct form and correct range of motion as well as working within your targeted work load.

Once you have good form and good range of motion with an exercise, you can consider what you want from your training. Do you want to be lean and strong with an athletic look? Do you want to be big and bulky like a bodybuilder or do you just want the strength?

A general rule of thumb is that if you want strength, you focus on low reps, heavy weight and a bigger number of sets. If you want to be lean and athletic, you focus on higher reps, which means, by default, you will lift lighter weights.

Here is a guide to help you decide on a workload zone that matches your goals:

General fitness: 3 sets of 12 - 15 reps

Strength training: 4 - 6 sets of 6 - 10 reps

Bodybuilding: 4 – 6 sets of 8 – 12 reps

Endurance: 3 – 6 sets of 25 – 50 reps

*** Please note that this does not include warm up sets. Warm up sets are performed with very low weight to get the joints and muscles ready for a "working set". One or two sets of the exercise performed with an empty bar or very light dumbbells at 15 – 20 reps is normal here.

As you can see, this workload guide is pretty diverse, but it should give you a good idea of the amount of sets and reps you should do per exercise.

All too often, there are frustrated trainers that aren't getting the results that they want from their exercise sessions, and this is normally one factor.

For example, "general fitness" falls into the category of weight loss and its very common to see people aiming for weight loss, but training in the "strength training" zone.

Another part of the workload is the actual resistance level or the weight being lifted. Ideally, we want to be training within our target workload zone but we also want to be challenging our muscles enough for development. During an exercise, if we can reach our targeted reps in a set easily, the weight is too light, an easy measure of this is that we want to be at 60% – 70% maximum effort or full exhaustion by the time we are hitting our final reps of the set.

In each workload zone listed, there is a range of sets and reps. For general fitness, we are aiming for 12 – 15 reps per set. So the first set could be with a lighter weight, if that is too easy, increase the weight for the next set and so on. This is known as pyramid training. To get the most out of this, it's an excellent idea to track your resistance level and reps completed in a notebook during your workouts.

Body positioning, exercise form and workload management are ongoing points for improvement and assessment. To sum this section up:

- Learn and understand the exercise
- Work to full range of movement on every rep
- Train within the workload dictated by your fitness goals
- Challenge yourself enough without sacrificing exercise form

Advanced Workload Option – One rep Max

The simplest way to understand how much resistance you need to be lifting for any type of progression is to train within your target reps and sets range and adjust the weight so you are close to failure at the end of each set. With compound exercises, however, if you are willing to put in a bit of extra work, you can test your "one rep max".

To do this, you will need to be fully warmed up. I would suggest a five to ten minutes steady state on a cross trainer or rower so that you get your joints and muscles ready for training. These cardio machines are perfect for warming up for a resistance workout, as they use most muscles in the body. A treadmill is still a viable choice, but this piece of equipment does not target the upper body's muscles as well as the other choices of cardio equipment.

Once you are warmed up, get set up for the compound exercise that you are testing your "one rep max" on. Let's use bench press as the example. First, perform a set of 12 reps bench press with just the bar, focus on the movement and make sure you are feeling the chest muscles through the movement. This set of 12 reps is to further warm up your muscles and joints to prepare for the working sets.

After this warm up set, add a weight to the bar that you know you can lift in good form and perform a single rep. Keep adding more weight to the bar and performing single reps with each increase of weight. You will get to a point where you can't lift the loaded bar in good form. Your one rep max for this exercise will be the weight that you could lift.

It's really important to focus on the muscle group that the compound exercise is designed to target. If you are focused on just moving the weight, your recorded one rep max might be inaccurate if you lose focus.

Bench press is a perfect example for me to share an experience of this in my training. My shoulders are stronger than my chest and shoulders are a synergist when performing bench press. So I can bench press a lot more weight than I should be able to. If I do this, however, my chest workout is diluted as my shoulders take over the lift. So If I were to test my one rep max on bench press, I would add plates to the bar, and perform single reps until I felt my shoulders kick in and felt the intensity on my chest diminish.

If I was focused on simply moving the bar from point A to point B, I could probably lift 20kg plus heavier than my true one rep max on bench press. But with bench press, I want to target my chest. The same principals apply to all other compound exercises.

My situation is probably different to others, so if you are testing your one rep max, have this in mind. The weight on the bar is not as important as the focus on the muscle you are training and the exercise form you are keeping.

Once you have your one rep max for each compound exercise, you can work out the resistance level you should train at for your working sets according to your fitness goals. Here are the workloads for each different fitness goal again, but with the added one rep max percentage:

General fitness: 3 sets of 12 - 15 reps @ **50% one rep max**

Strength training: 4 - 6 sets of 6 - 10 reps **@70% one rep max**

Bodybuilding: 4 – 6 sets of 8 – 12 reps **@85% one rep max**

Endurance: 3 – 6 sets of 25 – 50 reps **@60% one rep max**

Going back to the example of bench press, if we say that our one rep max was 40kg, this is the weight that we should work at for each different fitness goal:

General fitness: **50% one rep max = 20kg**

Strength training: **70% one rep max = 28kg**

Bodybuilding: **85% one rep max = 34kg**

Endurance: **60% one rep max = 24kg**

Working out your one rep max will give you a very good idea of the amount of resistance you should be training at, within your planned workload, dictated by your fitness goals.

When you work out your one rep max, it may not be convenient to work to it exactly. From our results above, it shows weight ranges that don't fit well to the usual weighted plates in most gyms. It's easier to work with multiples of five or ten, so if you find you have "28kgs" or "34kgs" for example, just round these up to "30kg" and "35kg".

As with most calculations in fitness and diet, this is just a guide to help you get the most out of your training and help you keep track of your progress. Everyone is different, but having a starting point, a unit of measure and a figure to track is far better than going in blind.

If you train consistently with a resistance routine, your body will adapt and you will become more capable of the workouts, so one rep max testing can be done every five to ten weeks. Your figures may change and you will have to adjust your working set resistance accordingly.

As mentioned in the opening part of this chapter, if you choose not to work out your one rep max for your compound exercises, which most people don't, you can still get the result that you want if you simply lift within your sets and reps range and gauge the resistance level by failure on the last rep of the set, you will challenge yourself enough, but maybe you have to reduce the resistance level for further sets of that exercise to reach the required number of reps needed for your goal. If this sounds familiar, it would be a massive benefit to plan in a few one rep max sessions.

A final thought on this and to reinforce the importance of correct workloads is that it's really common for a trainer to train in the wrong workload zone for their goal. If your training goal is for general fitness and fat loss, for example, but you have been lifting in the strength training zones, you will not get the best result for general fitness and fat loss, the training effect you will get will be strength.

Getting this right from the start will save a lot of frustration and will almost definitely get you the training results and progression much faster.

Types Of Barbell & Dumbbell Training

Barbells and dumbbell training can be fit into many different situations. It doesn't have to follow a set pattern of simple sets and reps, there are many training options. This section will cover some of the variety and situations you can choose to use these methods.

- **Sets & Reps**

"Sets and reps" has been covered earlier, but for clarity, "rep" is short for "repetition", meaning the amount of times we perform an exercise movement in our set. A set is the amount of times we perform a continued sequence of exercise movements before resting. Sets and reps can be used as a measure of our progress and to give us a guide that relates to our training goals.

- **Full Body Workouts**

Full body workouts are great for general fitness, endurance and foundation strength training. As the name suggests, this is a type of training that focuses on all major muscle groups in a single workout. This type of training is a great choice for trainers that have limited days to train on. Provided the workload and intensity is on point, full body workouts can lead to good progress with as little as three training sessions per week

- **Circuit Training**

Circuit training is a training method where several exercises are performed directly after each other. Normally, five or more exercises that target different muscle groups are added into a circuit and the amount of reps per set can vary. Circuit training is an excellent choice for trainers looking to reduce body fat percentage and tone muscle.

Because of the nature of this training method, designing a circuit for a specific goal can be a fun and creative task. There is a huge amount of scope for diversity with circuit training.

- **Split Training**

Split training is a great choice for bodybuilding and body shaping. Training with a split routine means that we split a training timeframe (usually a week) into several training routines based on muscle groups. A two-day split would mean that we may train chest, back and triceps on one day and biceps, legs, shoulders and abs on another day.

So we would have two workouts planned, a workout "A" and a workout "B". We would perform each one twice per week on consecutive days with a rest day between the four sessions, giving us three days to recover before hitting it again the next week.

- **Blitzing**

Blitzing is where we would focus on a single muscle group or body part in each workout. The idea is that we completely exhaust the focused muscle group with progressive overload. Blitzing is good for intermediate and advanced bodybuilding, but to achieve good progress and a balanced physique with this method, we will need more training sessions per week to cover all body parts, quality rest, and quality nutrition.

- ## Supersets

A superset is when we perform one set of two exercises back to back without a rest. Usually, the exercises would be on opposing body parts, such as biceps and triceps, or chest and back. A chest and back superset might look like this: 12 reps of bench press, followed immediately by 12 reps of bent over rows.

Supersets can be used for entire workouts, or for certain body parts. This training method is a good choice for trainers who would like to cut their workout time down, for bodybuilding, and for more advanced general fitness trainers.

- ## Drop sets

Drop sets are used to further exhaust a muscle group when failure has been reached in a regular set. Once the exercise can no longer be performed in good form due to fatigue, the resistance level is dropped and reps are continued. For example, we are performing a set of dumbbell shoulder press with the 20kg dumbbells and we manage to complete 10 good reps, but the 11th rep becomes impossible, to do a drop set, we would return the 20kg dumbbells and pick up the 12.5kg dumbbells and continue to exhaustion. There should be as little rest during the switch over as possible.

When it comes to deciding how much weight to drop per drop set, a good rule of thumb is to drop a 3rd of the weight on the bar.

Drop sets can be done as a single drop set; double of even a triple drop set, but this depends on the trainer and the training goal. Drop sets are great when using a blitzing routine and work well for bodybuilding.

- ## Pre exhaust

Pre exhaust sets are used to stimulate more muscle growth or to overcome a training plateau with growth or strength. Usually, several sets of an isolation exercise are performed on a muscle group working to target one of the major muscles in a compound movement. For example, lateral raises will be a pre exhaust exercise for shoulder press and leg extensions, leg curls or both will be pre exhaust sets for the compound exercise of squats.

The idea is that when your muscles are fatigued, they are forced to work harder to lift the big resistance that compound movements are known for. After a few weeks of pre exhaust sets, you will find that training fresh with compound movements, you will be able to increase the resistance level.

- Mixing it up

There is a lot of potential for every trainer and exercise doesn't have to be the same old grind. There's a lot we can do to make exercise interesting and more challenging and nobody said we have to stick to one training method, so if it fits with your fitness goals, mix it up a bit!

If you are looking for general fitness or fat loss and have three training days planned per week, why not design a full body circuit for one of your training days and have a 2 day split with simple sets and reps for the other two days?

If you are bodybuilding and want to try a two or three day split but have weaker areas that you would like to develop, why not design a split routine that uses blitzing for your weaker areas adding in drop sets?

There are situations where circuit training can be used in split routines, too. The more you train and get explore the options open to you, the more creative you will become. Although there are plenty of training options available, it's always important to make sure however you train, it should align with your overall fitness goals.

Mind & Muscle Connection

For any type of resistance training, exercise form is the number one priority. Getting the movement right before adding more resistance is a must. The next step is to actually focus on the muscles that the exercise is designed to target.

With bicep curls, we are targeting our biceps, with lateral raises we are targeting our lateral deltoids, and with big compound movements like squats, we are targeting our quads, glutes and hamstrings, and so on and so forth.

When we perform any exercise, there is always a target muscle or muscle group, therefore it's really important to understand the exercises that are in our routine.

Many people in the gym at some point, me included in the past, will approach a resistance workout or exercise with the view of just moving the weight from the start position to the finish position through a pre-planned amount of sets and reps. We are in the gym moving weights around, so the results will come, right? Yes, the results will come, but depending on the attention to detail of each rep, they could be significantly diluted.

To get the most out of every rep of every set, as well as making sure our exercise form is on point, we should also be focusing on the muscles that the exercise is targeting. This simply means that we are making sure we are actually using those muscles to perform each rep. It can take a lot of concentration, but it's worth every effort.

Along with the exercise illustrations in section 2, there will be a brief, written description that will clear this up for each exercise, but I'd like to look at an exercise in more depth here.

Let's look at barbell squats as an example:

First off, squats are not for everyone, but it's a big compound exercise that uses several large muscles to complete a single rep, so it serves as a great example.

This is the start position. The bar rests across our shoulders and is held in place with a grip that is comfortable (normally our hands would be just past shoulder width). We are standing with our feet just past shoulder width apart, toes pointing at a slight angle away from our bodys midline. We have a flat back, knees are not locked and we're looking forward.

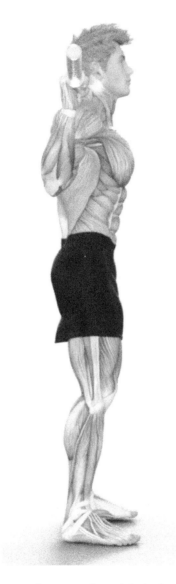

As we lower into the squat under control, we inhale, keeping our back flat and focus the workload towards our quads until we reach the "top of movement". Once at the top of the movement, we should pause slightly and prepare for the return. The reason for this pause for preparation is where the mind muscle connection is needed. The more used to this you become, the quicker you will be able to prepare, so the shorter the pause will be.

This is what the "top of movement looks like":

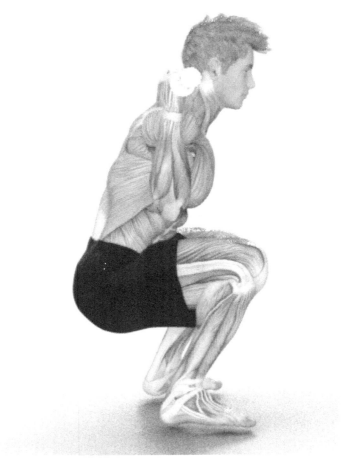

As you can see, we've maintained our upper body positioning until we get to our hips. Our pelvic tilt has moved slightly forward. On this, lower back problems can occur if the pelvic tilt is too exaggerated, and it's very natural to want to do this as a beginner to correct form squatting, but I believe this is due to lack of glute strength and/ or tight hip flexors. If squats are practiced correctly, glute and lower back strength will develop quickly, along with flexibility, in all working areas.

This "top of movement" position is where we pause and the preparation for return starts. Before we move, the first thing we should do is engage our glutes. To engage our glutes, we simply clench our butt cheeks together! You can try this right now. If you can't do it, there is something to work on.

Our quads will be engaged, as they will be taking most of the weight. We should take note of our knee position throughout the movement, but at the top of movement during our brief pause, we should ensure our knees are not tracking inwards. Our knees should be in line with our feet. This will ensure the full quad group is being used evenly and reduce stress on the knees.

With our glutes engaged and knees aligned, we maintain our flat back and head position and begin to exhale as we push through our heels to straighten the legs and return to the start position. We always push through our heels as this action transfers the workload to the quads and glutes while it also helps us to maintain a flat back and keep our form. If we push through the balls of our feet, the workload on the quads is diluted as the calve muscles kick in and we risk leaning forward, which can put a lot of stress on the lower back.

It may seem that the pause at the top of movement is a long one with all the things to consider, but with practice, this should take place in a second or two. And a good rule of thumb for each rep should be "two seconds up and two seconds down". This goes for all exercise choices.

Squat depth or the extent that we bend our knees is subjective. Ideally, we want to work to a full range of motion, but this is not possible for some and can be counterproductive to others. Because of some people's genetics, it can be difficult to squat lower than the point that their quads are parallel to the ground. This is normally with taller people. In these cases, quads being parallel to the ground is fine, but the optimum depth without putting too much stress on the knee is just past this point, as the illustration shows.

If you struggle with squat depth, it's a good idea to assess whether this is actually because of your makeup or whether it is down to lack of muscle strength or flexibility in certain areas. Try some body weight squats and look at your form in the mirror. Do you feel unstable? If so, what muscle group is making you feel this way? It may need some work.

This guide was not advertised to have a big emphasis on body mechanics, but approaching resistance training with an analytical mind-set in this area is always a big advantage. The more you put into practice what you learn about your body's strengths, weaknesses and ability, the more value you'll get out of your training.

Mind and muscle connection is an ongoing process. Hopefully, this breakdown of the squats exercise has highlighted what needs to be considered with every exercise that you choose to have in your workouts. Learning to engage and use the muscles that the exercise is designed to target goes hand in hand with practicing the correct form.

Basic Strength Training

Strength training is not just for strongman competitions, it's for everyone. Muscle strength is the foundation on which we build everything else, so muscle size and muscle tone will not come without building strength first. Even if your goal is to tone up and lose body fat, focus on strength training as a foundation.

It's fairly true to say that every resistance exercise builds strength, but there are some that offer us a far more efficient path to strength training and give us more potential for improvement.

First, I want to talk about the best exercise choices for strength training and why they are the best. Sure, you can build a certain amount of strength with exercises like lateral raises, dumbbell flys, tricep extensions and leg extensions, but these exercises are isolation exercises, meaning that they are designed to target a single muscle group.

Targeting a single muscle or muscle group with isolation exercises will, of course, develop a modicum of strength in that area, but on a rep to rep comparison with a compound exercise, the results will be increased significantly when training with compound exercises. The best exercises for strength training are exercises like bench press, squats, deadlift, rows and shoulder press. The most effective strength training routines will use these compound exercises.

The heavier you can lift with good form and within your target workload, the stronger you will become. Compound exercises give us the opportunity to lift heavier weights than isolation exercises, and they also use more than one muscle group at a time.

I'm a big believer in compound exercises and that they should be the bread and butter of most exercise routines. As long as we can perfect our form and push ourselves with this type of exercise, they should make up the majority of our training and be prioritised over other movements.

So to build strength and develop muscle, we need to lift heavy weights, but this does not have priority over exercise form. We also need to be lifting within our sets and reps range dictated by our goals mentioned in a previous chapter. When strength is our goal, we should aim at 4 - 6 sets of 6 - 10 reps.

When we take into consideration our exercise form and workload, we know we are lifting the correct weight when we are struggling to maintain our exercise form, because of the amount of resistance at around 6 reps. If we manage to perform 10 reps easily, we need to add more weight for the next set.

These workload ranges are only a guide, but have been effective for me and my clients in the past and I'm very aware that other trainers will have a slightly different theory, but the more you train, the more you will understand where your training sweet spot is. Your training sessions may be a bit messy at first, but if you are consistent with your training, within a few weeks you will have a good idea of the resistance that's most effective for you for each exercise. Try exercise sessions with 6 reps, then some with 10 reps, and see how you progress.

Performing compound exercises with barbells and dumbbells takes a lot more effort than performing isolation exercises. This is because we are using several large muscle groups during each rep, along with a whole bunch of stabiliser muscles and often with a heavier resistance level. For the beginner to resistance training, if training exclusively with compound exercises, gym sessions can be fairly minimal in order to get good results because of recovery time needed.

Beginners to weight training who are looking to lose body fat and tone muscle will often prioritise cardio training over resistance training and the resistance exercises that are chosen are isolation exercises or even abdominal workouts. Let's get this out of the way first; to lose fat; correct diet is the most effective condition, followed by calorie burning.

Training with compound exercises will burn a lot of calories, a lot more than training with isolation exercises. This calorie burning does not just happen when lifting the weights, it happens with recovery too. Simply put, lean muscle is a machine that uses fuel, so the more you have, the more fat you will be able to burn, even at rest. Training with compound exercises gives us the opportunity to burn more calories while lifting, as we are using much more energy to perform a single rep when compared to an isolation exercise and all of those muscles will work hard to recover.

So if your goal is fat loss and you want to add resistance training to your fitness routine, choose shoulder press over lateral raises, choose squats over leg extensions, choose chest press over flys, etc.

As a beginner, it's possible to train only twice or three times per week and still see good progress, depending on the muscle groups worked each training session. As we become more experienced, we will need to add more sessions to challenge our muscle groups more. To highlight this, there are several example routines in section 2 with explanations on when to use them and who they might be a good fit for.

It may appear that I'm biased towards compound exercises. This is probably true, but isolation exercises are actually still very valuable when used in the correct manner. This will also be highlighted in the example routines in section 2.

For some people, it may not be possible to perform certain exercises due to genetics or injury. Maybe back problems will impede our squatting ability, for instance, so barbell squats may be a no go. But if we have access to a gym, there are machines that simulate squats that protect the back, and these machines are still designed to perform compound movements, so this may be a way around a problem like this. If you find yourself in a situation like this, it can be extremely valuable to enlist the help of a physiotherapist to help you find ways to perform compound movements. I've mentioned in my other guides that working with a good physiotherapist can be game changing if you feel lost, but I'll mention it again here as in my experience, they can open a lot of doors.

Section 2

Exercise routines

If you are looking for results from your training, having a plan to follow is a must. Not only will it make life easier for you to keep track of, but it will give you better focus, you will know exactly what you are doing in the gym before you get there, it will save you a lot of time in the long run, it will give you accountability and you will be able to see where your strengths and weakness are.

The more focus you invest in this part of training, the better equipped you will be to change up your routine where it is needed. Although it's entirely plausible to start off with one of these routines right out of the book, it may not be the best fit for your personal circumstance. In this section, I aim to offer full routines, but also try to steer you towards creating something that's right for you and your goals.

There are many ways to create a fitness routine card, so this is not set in stone. The following cards are my design. The idea is to keep it simple, clear and present useful information about the training at a glance. There is also room for fluidity when updates need to be made.

Here is an example of a basic, blank training card. There will be multiple copies at the back of the book for you to fill in directly or make copies for personal use.

BARBELL & DUMBBELL TRAINING

FULL BODY ROUTINE

EXERCISE	SETS	REPS	RESISTANCE

WEEKS	MON	TUE	WED	THURS	FRI	SAT	SUN
1							
2							
3							
4							
5							

From this exercise card, we can fill in the exercises we plan to do, the sets and reps we plan to work to, the days we plan to train on and the resistance that we manage to lift with good form for each exercise we do. We can also plan for up to five weeks in advance for training sessions.

Generally speaking, in a five-week training timeline, we would not change the exercises or sets and reps we plan to work to, but we may change the training days and their frequency, so we can plan out and lock in the exercise choices we plan to train with and the sets and rep range we plan to work to as a start.

Depending on lifestyle, we may want to plan a single week of training at a time. If we have a set working life that won't change for the foreseeable future, we can go ahead and plan the full five weeks right away. If we find we are progressing quickly, we may want to change up the exercise frequency several weeks into our training plans. This is easily done on a week by week basis, so the training schedule may need regular reassessment.

The following program card shows a filled in version and is created for a beginner to resistance with a strength goal in mind.

Basic strength training

BARBELL & DUMBBELL TRAINING

FULL BODY BARBELL ROUTINE FOR STRENGTH TRAINING

EXERCISE	SETS	REPS	RESISTANCE
BARBELL CHEST PRESS	3	10	40kg
BENT OVER ROWS	3	10	30kg
SQUATS	3	10	40kg
BICEP CURLS	3	10	15kg
SHOULDER PRESS	3	10	20kg
SKULL CRUSHERS	3	10	10kg

WEEKS	MON	TUE	WED	THURS	FRI	SAT	SUN
1	*			*			
2	*			*			
3	*		*		*		
4	*		*		*		
5	*		*		*		

Who is this for?

This is for a beginner to develop a solid foundation in full body strength. Barbells may be more appropriate as there is slightly less to concentrate on with exercise form and this early training will help to develop stabiliser muscles. So I have advised on a full barbell training routine.

The exercise choices

The exercise choices have been chosen based on the trainer not having any physical issues; they are all compound exercises (apart from bicep and tricep movements) which are the best for strength training and a full body routine will challenge every major muscle group in each workout. Of course, you can add variations of these exercises to your plan or even add extra exercises in there too. But for a beginner, this is a solid start.

The sets and reps

Opting for 3 sets of 10 reps is a suitable start, as this range will challenge the trainer, and training on the higher end of the suggested strength range will allow more repetition to grow accustomed to the movement.

Training days

The first two weeks are set for two sessions per week, with an even gap in days between sessions. This should allow for suitable recovery between sessions. As these are full body workouts, this rest will be needed for a beginner or for someone who has been away from training for an extended period.

Depending on the individual, maybe these two training sessions per week will be needed for longer, but for this example, I have upped the frequency of sessions on the third week to highlight the possibilities. From week three to week five, there will be three training sessions per week, with even rest days between.

The resistance

Resistance or "weight lifted" is added in at the end of a training session or when the last set of an exercise has been finished. This is the variable that may change the most. When training for strength, we should always try to push ourselves, but never at the cost of exercise form. If this trainer managed to bench press 30 kg for 10 reps on their first set, 40kg for 10 reps on the second set and then manage to get 9 good reps for the third set with 45kg. For this trainer, as a beginner, I would suggest that "40kg" is written in the resistance column. A more experienced trainer may be working within a rep range, so could record the resistance of the third set.

The resistance may fluctuate from session to session, so this column can be updated regularly. Some muscle groups may develop quicker than others, and this is part of identifying your strengths and weaknesses.

Here's an example to show what a "working" card may look like. Take note of the "resistance" column.

BARBELL & DUMBBELL TRAINING

FULL BODY BARBELL ROUTINE FOR STRENGTH TRAINING

EXERCISE	SETS	REPS	RESISTANCE
BARBELL CHEST PRESS	3	10	40kg
BENT OVER ROWS	3	10	~~30kg~~ 40kg
SQUATS	3	10	~~40kg~~ ~~50kg~~ 70kg
BICEP CURLS	3	10	~~15kg~~ 20kg
SHOULDER PRESS	3	10	~~20kg~~ 25kg
SKULL CRUSHERS	3	10	10kg

WEEKS	MON	TUE	WED	THURS	FRI	SAT	SUN
1	*			*			
2	*			*			
3	*		*		*		
4	*		*		*		
5	*		*		*		

46

Full body split training

It's perfectly possible to cut down on workout time and increase workout sessions while still training with the same exercises. A split routine is simply training several body parts in different training sessions.

Here is an example of the previous routine made into a 2 day split routine:

BARBELL & DUMBBELL TRAINING

FULL BODY BARBELL ROUTINE FOR STRENGTH TRAINING 2 DAY SPLIT

EXERCISE	SETS	REPS	RESISTANCE
WORKOUT "A"			
BARBELL CHEST PRESS	3	10	~~30kg~~ 40kg
BENT OVER ROWS	3	10	40kg
SKULL CRUSHERS	3	10	10kg
WORKOUT "B"			
BICEP CURLS	3	10	~~15kg~~ 20kg
SQUATS	3	10	~~40kg~~ ~~50kg~~ 70kg
SHOULDER PRESS	3	10	~~20kg~~ 25kg

WEEKS	MON	TUE	WED	THURS	FRI	SAT	SUN
1	A			B			
2	A			B			
3	A		B		A		
4	B		A		B		
5	A	B		A	B		

As you can see, the exercises have been split over two sessions. We have an "A" day and a "B" day.

Routine A

In routine "A" we are still doing 3 sets of 10 reps, but in this session we are only doing three exercises. Barbell bench press for chest, bent over rows for back and skull crushers for triceps.

Routine B

In routine "B" we are also still doing 3 sets of 10 reps with three exercises, but we have Bicep curls for biceps, squats for legs and shoulder press for shoulders.

Deciding how to split this routine

There are no rules as to which body parts you decide to train in each split, but you can make decisions based on the exercises you have. For example, I chose to put the back exercise in a different session than the leg exercise. The idea is that these are two big muscle groups and it might make the session less intense, so when these muscle groups are trained, they will have better focus.

I also decided to put tricep exercises with chest as with the exercise chest press. The triceps are a synergist, so they will have extra intensity and may develop better. There was also an opportunity to add biceps to the back exercise as biceps are a synergist to bent over rows, but I didn't want to put biceps and triceps in the same session.

If you are planning your workout and have the same issue, a good idea is to decide whether your biceps or triceps need more work. Once you decided, you could put the muscle group that needs more work into a session where it will be used as a synergist.

Workout days

At the bottom of the card you will see that instead of check marks in the training days, we have either an "A" or a "B". Weeks 1 and 2, we are training with "A" on Monday and "B" on Thursday. This means that we are still training the same body parts as in the full body routine, but over 2 days.

An upgrade to this is working out every other week day but switching from "A" to "B" each session and this carries over to the following upgrade, which turns into a four session week. At this point, we are training each muscle group twice per week.

Again, there are many ways to set this up, and this example may not be typical of progression, it may be that you stick at two sessions per week for longer or it may be that you bump it up to four sessions per week sooner. Hopefully, this gives you some ideas about what is possible.

The exercises and workload on these examples are geared towards beginner strength training, so the goal here is to build a good foundation in strength over the full body. But just because these exercises are some of the best for strength training, doesn't mean that they can only be used for this fitness goal.

If we tweak the workload, we can use the same exercise routine for general fitness and fat loss. All we have to do it to increase the rep range from 3 sets of 10 reps to 4 sets of 15 reps.

Doing this will affect the amount of resistance we can lift for a set, but as we are working for longer, we are burning more calories and adding more intensity to the working sets.

The same routine for general fitness, body toning and fat loss may look like this:

FULL BODY BARBELL ROUTINE FOR FAT LOSS AND MUSCLE TONE

EXERCISE	SETS	REPS	RESISTANCE
BARBELL CHEST PRESS	3	15	30kg
BENT OVER ROWS	3	15	20kg
SQUATS	3	15	30kg
BICEP CURLS	3	15	15kg
SHOULDER PRESS	3	15	15kg
SKULL CRUSHERS	3	15	7.5kg

WEEKS	MON	TUE	WED	THURS	FRI	SAT	SUN
1	*			*			
2	*			*			
3	*		*		*		
4	*		*		*		
5	*		*		*		

All that has changed here is that we have changed the amount of reps we are performing in each exercise. We still want to be working with a resistance that challenges us, so to gauge this; we should be near failure on the last few reps.

This is a simple way to ensure we are working at enough intensity to get results. There are ways of testing our "1 rep max" and working at a percentage of this, but this figure can change quickly, depending on the trainer. So as long as we maintain good exercise form, are targeting the muscles that we are supposed to be working and we are challenging ourselves with each set in our workload range, we will progress.

It's very common to want to add more resistance to an exercise at the expense of exercise form. If you find yourself in a position where you know you've added more than you can handle, just strip it back and start the set again. There is no harm in trying to increase weight on the bar, but if it's too heavy, you risk "just moving weight around" meaning that the set is nowhere near as valuable as it would be with a lighter weight. This goes for strength training, fat loss training and bodybuilding and body toning.

The last example of a workout that I want to share is a 2 day split bodybuilding routine. Here's the routine:

BARBELL & DUMBBELL TRAINING			
BODYBUILDING 2 DAY SPLIT TRAINING 2 DAY SPLIT			
EXERCISE	SETS	REPS	RESISTANCE
WORKOUT "A"			
DB FLYS	4	12	
BARBELL CHEST PRESS	4	12	
DB PULLOVERS	4	12	
BENT OVER ROWS	4	12	
SKULL CRUSHERS	4	12	
CRUNCHES	4	RF	
WORKOUT "B"			
BICEP CURLS	4	12	
LUNGES	4	12	
SQUATS	4	12	
STIFF LEG DEADLIFT	4	12	
LATERAL RAISES	4	12	
SHOULDER PRESS	4	12	

WEEKS	MON	TUE	WED	THURS	FRI	SAT	SUN
1	A	B		A	B		
2	A	B		A	B		
3	A	B		A	B		
4	A	B		A	B		
5	A	B		A	B		

Who is this for?

This is a routine that's aimed at the beginner to intermediate bodybuilder. Before a routine like this is used, I would always advise that a basic strength routine is followed for at least four weeks. If we have a good foundation in strength training, this routine is a great upgrade, as it will take things to the next level, adding extra intensity and workload. The body will adapt to this type of training a lot easier if it has strength training experience.

The exercise choices

There are countless ways to create a 2 day split, so this is not the definitive answer by any means, but here is the theory behind my exercise choices. In this example, I've chosen to split the body into the same muscle groups as in the previous 2 day split for the same reasons. The difference is that we now have more than a single exercise for each muscle group.

The first exercise for a muscle group in this example is used as a "pre exhaust" movement. This is usually an isolation exercise and, as the name suggests, it's designed to exhaust the muscle before the big compound movement. This means that the muscles are working harder throughout the session, so we have the opportunity for more progression.

Routine "A"

We have DB flys, designed to pre exhaust the chest muscles before a doing bench press, we have DB pullovers, designed to pre exhaust the lats (back muscles) before doing bent over rows, skull crushers to work the triceps and we finish with some crunches for our abs.

Routine "B"

We have bicep curls, lunges to pre exhaust the quads before squats, stiff leg deadlifts to hit the hamstrings, lateral raises to pre exhaust the shoulders before shoulder press. Abs can be added to this routine too at the end if you feel the need.

The sets and reps

As this is a bodybuilding routine, I have chosen 4 sets of 12 reps for the workload for all exercises apart from the abs exercises. The rep range for abs can be to "RF" which stands for "reasonable failure". With reasonable failure, we are aiming to complete as many reps as possible before we exhaust our abdominals. You may find with reasonable failure that your first set is significantly higher than the rest. This is normal.

Training days

I have chosen to train on Mondays, Tuesdays, Thursdays and Fridays, alternating routine A with routine B throughout. This means we are training each body part twice per week. The other days can be total rest days, cardio days or even abs and calf days, depending on your goals, but rest is important, especially if you are newer to resistance training, so this is something to consider when creating your own routine.

The resistance

The resistance level will be dictated by your current ability and progression. It's worth noting that the pre exhaust exercises do not need to be as intense as the compound exercises, although you should still challenge your muscle group with isolations. I would suggest that when training with pre exhaust sets, that you work at 80% of your max rep range. For example, if you can perform an isolation exercise with a 10kg dumbbell for 12 reps and are at failure by the 12th rep, drop the weight to an 8kg dumbbell. This way, you have still challenged your muscle group enough to pre-exhaust it because of the rep range and set volume, but you are not at failure, so the reps that are performed will be good quality.

Once the muscles are used to this type of training, you can experiment with higher weights.

Circuit Training

Circuit training is an excellent method of training for muscle tone, fat loss and cardio. In fact, it is my go to fitness method for intermediate clients wanting this result. It is very plausible for a total beginner to start with circuit training, as I know many other trainers use this method exclusively. But I would suggest that a basic strength training routine was used for at least four weeks before jumping into circuit training.

A barbell and dumbbell circuit can get very tough, very quickly depending on the exercises used and the placement of these exercises. Fatigue is the biggest culprit in loss of good exercise form, and this is not what we want!

There are two main reasons that I would suggest a basic strength training routine is used beforehand, the first being the familiarisation of the exercise. If we are used to performing a certain exercise, learning the correct position, how it feels and the amount of resistance we can safely lift, this will not only get us ready for using this exercise within a circuit, but it will prepare our muscles and joints correctly, so we can get the most out of this more intense method of fitness.

Because of the nature of circuit training, during the workout, our heart rate will be higher for an extended time, which is why it's a superb choice for fat burning and developing stamina. Stamina is a big part of circuit training and even though strength training is not geared towards this goal, there will still be an element of stamina gained from a basic strength training routine that will prepare us as beginners to progress to a circuit. So earning this base level of stamina from strength training by default is our second reason for not jumping right into circuits.

What is circuit training?

Circuit training is a method of training where we perform one set of an exercise and move immediately on to another using at least five exercises. Because circuit training is designed for muscle tone, fat loss and general fitness, we should perform 12-15 reps of each exercise.

Which exercises can I use for circuit training?

You can use any exercises for circuit training. The whole body can be targeted in a circuit. You can even design a 2 day split with circuit training. It's important to remember that compound exercises take a lot more effort to perform than isolation exercises, so the toughest circuits will be the ones which exclusively use compound movements.

Which order do I perform the exercises in?

There is a fair bit of debate about this, but here's my take: You should have exercises that target smaller muscle groups at the start and end of the circuit and exercises that target the bigger muscle groups in the middle. If you are adding an abdominal or lower back exercise, these should always be at the end of the circuit.

Although the circuit gets harder with each exercise performed, having exercises that target smaller muscle groups first and last with the bigger exercises in the middle will create a gentler curve in intensity. If you imagine travelling around a 400m track, you will start off jogging, sprint in the middle and finish off by jogging. I have always preferred this way of exercising, as it feels kinder on the body.

The argument against this is that if you perform the exercises that target the bigger muscle groups first, you will be able to perform them better, and these are the exercises that have the most impact on results, but going back to the 400m track, this would represent sprinting for the first part and jogging for the middle and last part.

I'll leave this up to you to ponder over; it might even be worth trying it out and seeing which you prefer. As I said, there are a few different takes on this and what works for some might not work for others.

Here is an example of a full body circuit training routine using both compound and isolation exercises:

FULL BODY CIRCUIT ROUTINE BEGINNER

EXERCISE	REPS	RESISTANCE	SETS
BICEP CURLS	12		
LATERAL RAISES	12		
SQUATS	12		
BENT OVER ROWS	12		
SKULL CRUSHERS	12		
CHEST PRESS	12		
CRUNCHES	RF		3

WEEKS	MON	TUE	WED	THURS	FRI	SAT	SUN
1	*		*		*		
2	*		*		*		
3	*		*		*		
4	*		*		*		
5	*		*		*		

Who is this for?

This is designed for a beginner/ intermediate trainer who is familiar with the exercise choices and looking to burn fat, tone muscle and improve stamina with a full-body workout routine.

The exercise choices

I've chosen to use isolation exercises for the biceps, shoulders and triceps as these are smaller muscle groups and chosen to add compound exercises for the legs and back, and finally I've added an abdominal exercise at the end.

As you can see, the compound exercises for the big muscle groups are in the middle of the circuit and the isolation exercises are at the beginning and end.

The sets and reps

As this is for a beginner, the reps for each exercise are set at 12 and the sets or "circuits" are set at 3.

To perform a single circuit, we will perform 12 reps of each exercise immediately after the previous, starting with bicep curls and finishing on crunches. Once we have finished our crunches, we have completed a single circuit.

A note on crunches reps – Crunches can be performed until "reasonable failure" or "RF". This means that you perform as many as you can while maintaining good form and connection with the muscle. As soon as you can no longer feel your abs working or become fatigued, this is your "RF" point.

Training days

This routine will work well for a beginner or intermediate trainer being performed three times per week. If you decide to follow this and find that it's not challenging enough, you can add an extra training day or increase the amount of sets or "circuits you do".

The resistance

I've left the resistance blank here, as this will be based on the individual. The easy way to gauge this is to use a resistance level where failure is at the 12th rep. But if you would like to ensure you are working to a challenging level for your circumstance, use 50% of your 1 rep max on the compound movements as explained in an earlier section.

Rest between circuits

Rest between circuits is again something that will vary from trainer to trainer. I have found that around the 2 minute mark is a good starting point for a rest period. But this depends on the trainer. Ideally, you want to be in a situation where your breathing is back to normal and any lactic acid build-up has gone, but you don't want to have cooled down completely. A tip between circuits is to stay standing up, be thinking about the next circuit, stretch out the muscles you have worked and start to regulate your breathing as soon as you finish a set.

Final thoughts on circuit training

Circuit training has a high level of versatility to it. If you want to try this exclusively, you can plan a single circuit that can be repeated, or plan several that you can train with on different days. For progression, think about:

- Changing the amount of sets (circuits) in your workout
- Increasing the reps per exercise
- Increasing the resistance level
- Increasing the amount of exercises
- Training certain muscle groups in each circuit
- Creating a compound exercise only circuit
- Shorten the rest period between circuits

There are blank program cards at the back of the book for you to copy and use for your personal use if you would like to create your own circuit training routines.

The Exercises

Section 3

Introduction to section 3

Here, you will find a range of exercise choices using barbells and dumbbells. There are at least two illustrations of each exercise that show the starting position and end position of each movement. These illustrations also show correct posture, form and have written descriptions that detail how to perform the exercise correctly.

Posture and exercise form, during exercise, is extremely important, so please have this at the forefront of your mind when practicing and performing all exercises.

Along with the illustration of each exercise, there is a description. If you are new to a certain movement, it's best to have a go at the exercises and make sure you can perform it correctly before getting into the actual workouts.

If you are creating your own exercise routine, there are some blank exercise cards for you to fill in at the back of the book.

Chest exercises

Barbell flat bench press

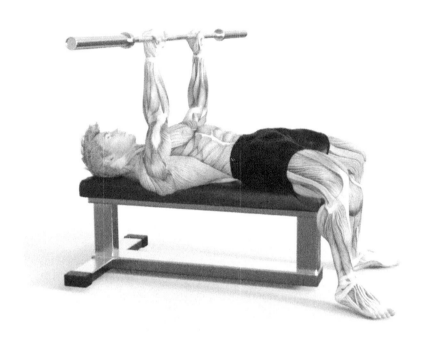

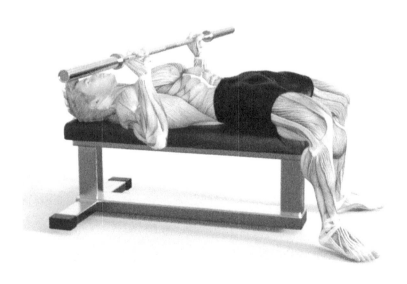

Start position

- This exercise is a compound movement for the mid chest
- Select a flat bench under a racked bar if possible
- Grip the barbell so that your hands are slightly wider than shoulder width apart
- Arms should be extended in front of you with a slight bend in the elbow
- Back should be flat on the bench and feet flat on the floor

Movement

- As you inhale, lower the bar to your mid-chest under control
- Lower to where you feel the stretch across the chest
- Once at the top of movement, exhale as you return to the start position

Extra info

It's common for trainers to have a slightly different elbow flare on a bench press than others because of their body mechanics. Ideally, elbows should only flare out slightly when the bar is lowered.

Barbell incline bench press

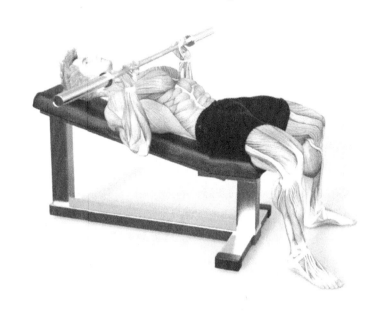

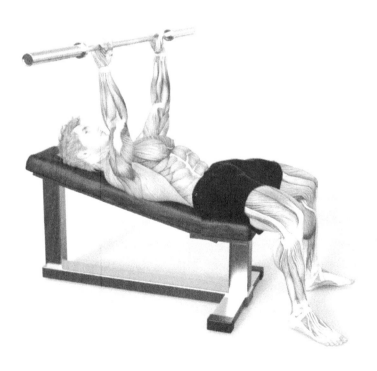

Start position

- This is a compound movement for the upper chest
- Select an incline bench underneath a racked bar if possible
- Back flat on the bench, feet flat on the floor
- Grip the barbell so that your hands are slightly wider than shoulder width apart
- Ensure that your arms are fully extended but maintain a slight bend at the elbows

Movement

- As you inhale, lower the bar towards your upper chest
- You should only lower to where you feel the stretch
- Once at the top of movement, as you exhale, return to the start position

Extra info

When setting up an incline bench, it's only necessary to have a slight incline. Many benches are adjustable and can be moved to an incline in increments. If you have one of these, normally, only two increments towards an incline are needed. The higher you move the bench on the incline, the more the chest workout is diluted in favour of the shoulder muscles.

Barbell decline bench press

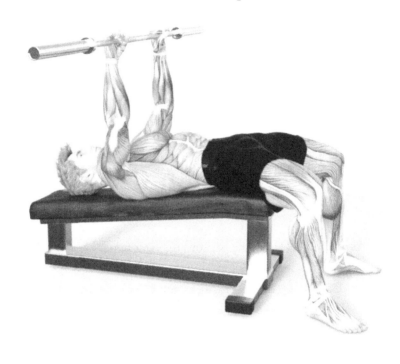

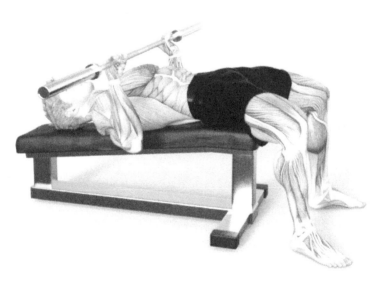

Start position

- This is a compound movement for the lower chest
- Select a decline bench underneath a racked bar if possible
- Grip the barbell so that your hands are slightly wider than shoulder width apart
- Your arms should be fully extended with a slight bend in the elbows and the bar should be above your lower chest
- Keep your back flat on the bench
- Keep your feet flat to the floor or use the benches foot pads if it has them

Movement

- Inhale as you lower the bar towards your lower chest
- Lower only to where you feel the stretch
- Take care not to flare your elbows too much as you lower
- Once at the top of movement, exhale as you return to the start position

Extra info

When selecting a bench for decline exercises, only a small increment towards the decline position is necessary. There are pieces of optional kit that are designed for decline exercises as foot anchors. Adjustable benches can often facilitate foam pads that attach to the foot of the bench to make decline exercises more comfortable and offer security against slipping.

Flat dumbbell flys

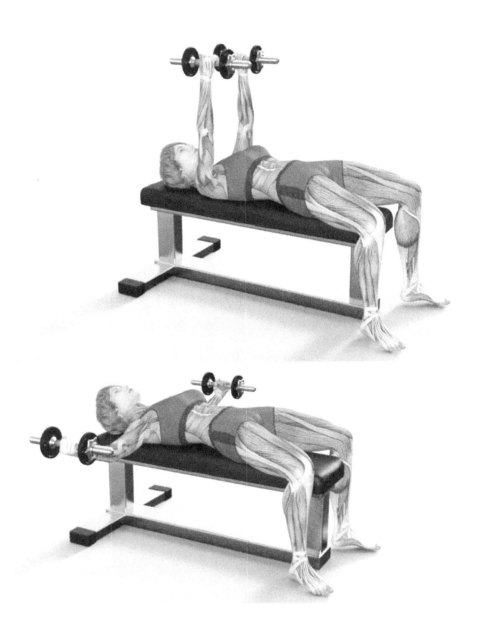

Start position

- This is an isolation exercise for the mid chest
- Select a flat bench and the correct set of dumbbells for your set
- Sit on the bench with the dumbbells on your quads
- As you lay back, bring the dumbbells back with your upper body
- Push the dumbbells up until your arms are fully extended with a slight bend in the elbows
- The dumbbells should be above your mid-chest, palms facing inwards
- Back flat on the bench and feet flat on the floor

Movement

- As you inhale, lower the dumbbells to your sides
- Ensure that your elbows are locked in a slightly bent position
- Ensure that your arms lower directly in line with your mid chest
- Lower only to where you feel the stretch
- As you exhale, return to the start position

Extra info

When performing this exercise, the dumbbells should stay stable and not rotate.

Incline dumbbell flys

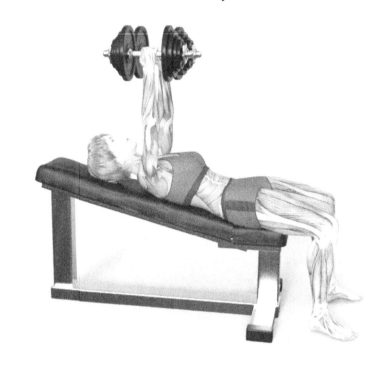

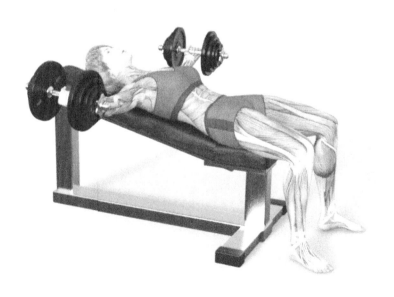

Start position

- This is an isolation exercise for the upper chest
- Select a slightly incline bench and the correct set of dumbbells for your set
- Sit on the bench with the dumbbells on your quads
- As you lay back, bring the dumbbells back with your upper body
- Push the dumbbells up until your arms are fully extended with a slight bend in the elbows
- The dumbbells should be above your upper chest, palms facing inwards
- Back flat on the bench and feet flat on the floor

Movement

- As you inhale, lower the dumbbells to your sides
- Ensure that your elbows are locked in a slightly bent position
- Ensure that your arms lower directly in line with your upper chest
- Lower only to where you feel the stretch
- As you exhale, return to the start position

Extra info

When performing this exercise, the dumbbells should stay stable and not rotate

Decline dumbbell flys

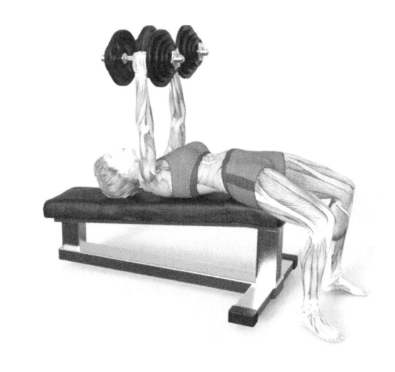

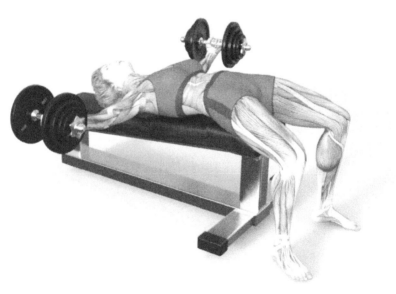

Start position

- This is an isolation exercise for the lower chest
- Select a bench with a slight decline and the correct set of dumbbells for your set
- Sit on the bench with the dumbbells on your quads
- As you lay back, bring the dumbbells back with your upper body
- Push the dumbbells up until your arms are fully extended with a slight bend in the elbows
- The dumbbells should be above your lower chest, palms facing inwards
- Back flat on the bench and feet flat on the floor or hooked around an attachment if you have one

Movement

- As you inhale, lower the dumbbells to your sides
- Ensure that your elbows are locked in a slightly bent position
- Ensure that your arms lower directly in line with your lower chest
- Lower only to where you feel the stretch
- As you exhale, return to the start position

Extra info

If this is a new exercise, be aware of your arm positioning when lowering. It's common to bring the arms closer to the head, as the position can be slightly disorienting. Arms going closer to the head will cause the lower chest tension to be diluted

Back exercises

Barbell bent over rows regular grip

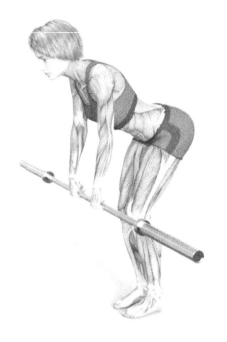

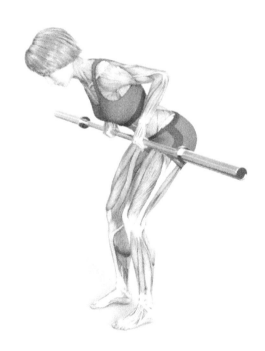

Start position

- This is a compound exercise for the back muscles
- Pick up a bar with a grip that places your hands about shoulder width apart
- Bend your knees slightly
- Keep your back flat and hinge at the hips so your upper body is set at about 45 degrees to the floor
- Straighten your arms but keep a slight bend in the elbows
- The bar should hang in this position in line with your lower abdominals

Movement

- As you exhale, pull the bar towards your belly button
- Keep your back flat and glutes engaged
- Focus on pushing your chest forward and your shoulders back
- Keep your elbows towards your body's midline
- Inhale as you return to the start position

Extra info

It is possible to perform this exercise with your upper body at a right angle to the floor, but in my experience, this puts more strain on the lower back, so 45 degrees is preferable. When bringing the bar towards your body, remember to maintain a flat back.

Barbell bent over rows close grip

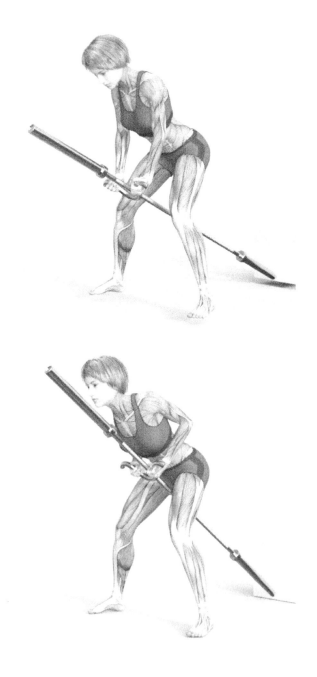

Start position

- This is a compound exercise for the back muscles
- Select a bar that has a close grip attachment
- Grip the bar so that your hands are close to your body's midline
- Bend your knees slightly and place your feet just past shoulder width
- Keep your back flat and hinge at the hips so your upper body is set at about 45 degrees to the floor
- Straighten your arms but keep a slight bend in the elbows
- The bar should hang in this position in line with your lower abdominals

Movement

- As you exhale, pull the bar towards your belly button
- Keep your back flat and glutes engaged
- Focus on pushing your chest forward and your shoulders back
- Keep your elbows towards your body's midline
- Inhale as you return to the start position

Extra info

Although this exercise shows an Olympic bar secured against a wall and an attachment that places the grip with the palms facing inwards, there are several ways to perform it. You may have access to different attachments that allow you to use a regular grip. There is also an opportunity to try an under hand grip too, but which ever variant you decide to use in your workouts, the movement is the same.

Dumbbell pullovers

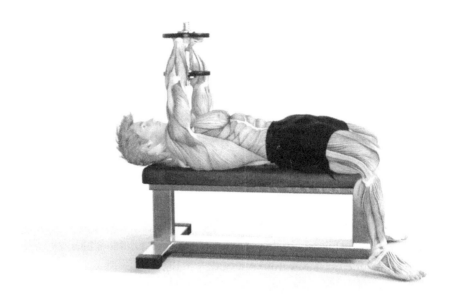

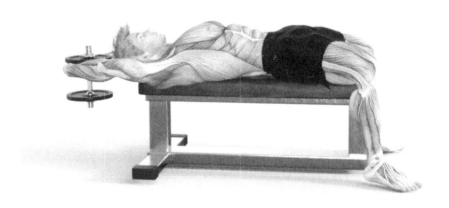

Start position

- This is an isolation exercise for the back muscles
- Select a flat bench and a single dumbbell that's right for you
- Sit on the bench with the dumbbells bottom plate resting on your quads
- Place your hands so they overlap on the inside of the bottom plate of the dumbbell
- Your fingers should be above the bar and thumbs underneath it
- As you lay back on the bench, tilt the dumbbell to follow your upper body
- Push the dumbbell above your chest so your arms are fully extended with a slight bend in the elbows and elbows should be slightly flared
- Feet flat on the floor, head slightly over the end of the bench and back pressed into the bench

Movement

- As you inhale, lower the dumbbell back above your head to where you feel the stretch in your lats
- Once at the top of the movement, exhale as you return to the start position
- Ensure you keep your elbows slightly flared and locked with the slight bend you started with

Extra info

This can be a tricky exercise to perfect. Flaring your elbows is important for targeting the back muscles. If you turn your elbows on, your chest will engage. Some trainers find that bending the elbows a bit more along with the flare helps to hit the lats more for them. If you have trouble with this exercise, try using a lighter dumbbell and experiment with differing levels of elbow flare and bend.

Dumbbell single arm rows

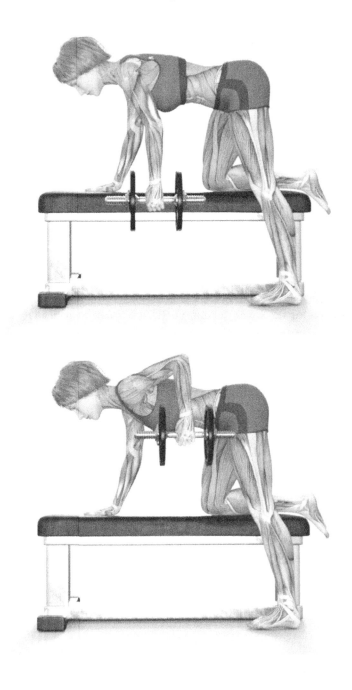

Start position

- This is a compound exercise for the back muscles
- Select a flat bench and a single dumbbell that's right for your workload
- Kneel on the bench with one leg and place the other foot flat on the floor
- Hinge at the hips and place the hand of your kneeling leg flat on the bench in line with your knee
- Your back should be flat aligned with your neck and head
- Pick up the dumbbell with your free hand. It should be directly beneath your shoulder

Movement

- As you exhale, pull the dumbbell up towards your lower abdominals
- Keep your back flat, hand and knee firmly on the bench and head in a neutral position
- Your elbow should be kept in towards your side and the dumbbell should not rotate
- Once at the top of movement, return to the start position as you inhale

Extra info

Once you have connected with this movement, you can actually start from a lower position to get a bigger extension of the back muscles. This works by tilting your body to the side of the dumbbell so you technically increase the range of motion. If you reach this point, it's important that even though you are tilting your body, you ensure you keep a flat back and neutral head position.

Deadlift

Barbell deadlift

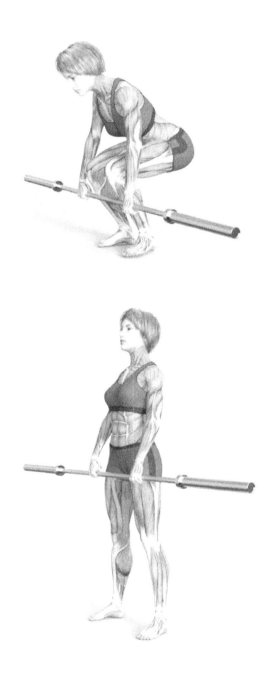

Start position

- This is a compound exercise for the back and legs
- Select a straight bar and stand in the middle with your toes underneath
- Your legs should be about shoulder width apart with your toes slightly turned out
- Squat down and take an overhand grip with your hands so they are outside your knees
- Keep your back flat and head in a neutral position
- Your feet should be flat on the floor

Movement

- Before you lift, ensure that your elbows are slightly bent and locked in this position
- Engage your glutes and abdominals
- As you exhale, stand up with the bar, keeping it close to your body and pull your shoulders back
- Once at the top of the movement, inhale and return to the start position

Extra info

A few points on deadlift; you might hear of an "alternate grip" (one hand overhand and the other underhand). This is ok, but is only used for very heavy lifts to help guard against loss of grip. A common injury from a deadlift is a bicep tear. There is more chance of a bicep tear from using an underhand grip.

The next point is hyper extending the back at the top of movement. Trainers use this to hit the lower back, again a technique that is plausible, but the lower back is part of the posterior chain so it will be worked from engaging the glutes in the start position.

As deadlifts are a big movement, there is a lot to concentrate on and a lot can go wrong, so please perfect the basic technique first, before experimenting with other methods mentioned if you feel the need to go down this route.

I always advise against underhand grip and hyper-extending, but I'm just one trainer and I know others will have differing opinions', It's best to explore these and follow the advice that seems most logical to you while considering your training goals, physical condition and weighing up the pros and cons.

Barbell sumo Deadlift

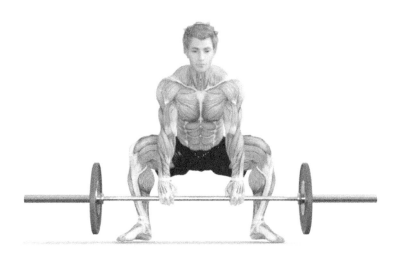

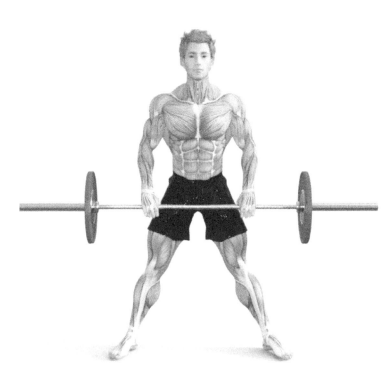

Start position

- This is a compound exercise for the back and legs
- Select a straight bar and stand in the middle with your toes underneath
- Your legs should be wider than shoulder width apart with your toes should be in line with your knees
- Squat down and take an overhand grip with your hands so they are inside your knees
- Keep your back flat and head in a neutral position
- Your feet should be flat on the floor

Movement

- Before you lift, ensure that your elbows are slightly bent and locked in this position
- Engage your glutes and abdominals
- As you exhale, stand up with the bar, keeping it close to your body and pull your shoulders back
- Once at the top of the movement, inhale and return to the start position

Extra info

Everything mentioned about the lift in the regular deadlift applies here, too. The sumo deadlift is slightly different because it targets the glutes and hamstrings that bit more. Have an experiment with the position. It's best to start off with a narrower stance until you are comfortable with the movement before going wider.

Dumbbell deadlift

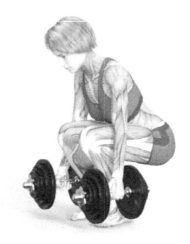

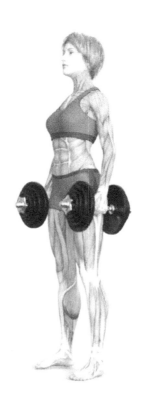

Start position

- This is a compound exercise for the back and legs
- Select a set of dumbbells and place them on the floor on the outside of your feet
- Your legs should be about shoulder width apart with your toes slightly turned out, following the line of your knees
- Squat down and grip the bars of the dumbbells, palms facing inwards
- Keep your back flat and head in a neutral position
- Your feet should be flat on the floor

Movement

- Before you lift, ensure that your elbows are slightly bent and locked in this position
- Engage your glutes and abdominals
- As you exhale, stand up with the dumbbells, keeping them close to your outer legs and pull your shoulders back
- Once at the top of the movement, inhale and return to the start position

Extra info

Using dumbbells for deadlift is not as common as using barbells, but it's still a great choice. It can be uncomfortable for some trainers, as the dumbbells have a tendency to knock on the legs, depending on the width of the stance. If you are lucky enough to have access to a "trap bar", you can simulate this movement without this problem.

Leg exercises

Barbell squats

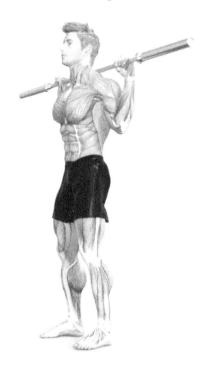

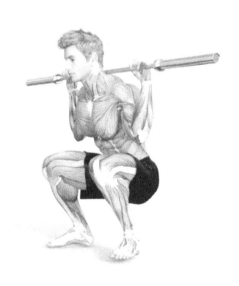

Start position

- This is a compound movement for the leg muscles
- Select a straight bar, preferably on a rack that is just below shoulder height
- Stand underneath the bar so that it rests across your trapezius and shoulder muscles
- Take the weight by straightening your legs whilst keeping your back flat and head in a neutral position
- Take a step back from the rack and set your feet so they are about shoulder width apart, toes slightly turned out and in line with your knees
- Keep a slight bend in your knees

Movement

- Before you start the movement, take a deep breath, engage your glutes and abdominals
- When ready, squat down by bending at the knees as if you were aiming to sit on a bench
- Your glutes will lead your upper body towards the floor
- Once your upper legs are parallel to the floor, this is the top of movement
- At this point, return to the start position by driving through your mid foot. Driving through your heels will put more emphasis on the quads
- Once you have finished your set, walk the bar back to the rack

Extra info

Squats are a fantastic exercise for all types of fitness, but as it's a big lift and there is a lot to think about, practice is needed. There are common mistakes with the squat, which include bending at the hips; this will cause a lot of undue strain on the lower back, so keep the alignment as you squat. Another mistake is heels rising off the floor during the movement. If this happens, the workload is being taken away from the quads and glutes and put onto the calfs. If you find this is the case, practice the squat but on set up, concentrate on planting your feet with your weight pushing through your heels. Raising the heels during a squat can be due to lack of strength in the glutes, but it can also be a confidence thing. Try putting a bench between your legs during your squat. If it's a confidence thing, you will soon get over it.

Squat depth is another debatable issue. Squatting to a depth where your upper legs are parallel to the ground is safe for most people, but some have the genetic makeup to perform a slightly deeper squat without problems. A deeper squat will work the quads through a bigger range of motion, but it will put more strain on the knees.

Barbell stiff leg deadlift

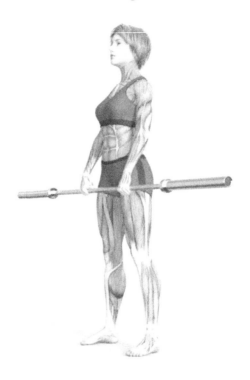

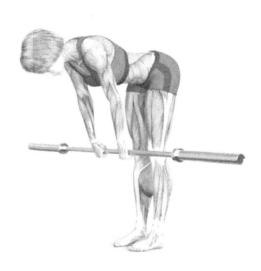

Start position

- This is an isolation exercise for the hamstrings and glutes
- Select a straight bar. Take an overhand grip of the bar with hands just outside shoulder width apart
- Arms should be fully extended with a slight bend in the elbows and the bar should hang close to the body
- Stand with your feet about hip width apart with your toes pointing forward
- Ensure that your back is flat and head is in a neutral position
- Keep a slight bend in the knees throughout this exercise

Movement

- Before you start the movement, engage your glutes
- As you exhale, hinge at the hips to lower your upper body towards the floor, keeping the bar close to your body
- Keep your back flat and head in a neutral position
- Lower to the point where you feel the stretch in your hamstrings
- Once at the top of the movement, inhale as you return to the start position

Extra info

Although this is called a "Stiff leg deadlift", having a slight bend in the knees will help to protect the knee joints, so have this in mind when performing the exercise. The foot position can be changed with this exercise. It's common to perform stiff leg deadlift with the feet together and pointing forward, this is fine.

Engaging your glutes before you start this exercise will help to strengthen your lower back while also minimising the risk of back pain. Keeping the bar close to your body will also mitigate this risk further.

Barbell sumo squat

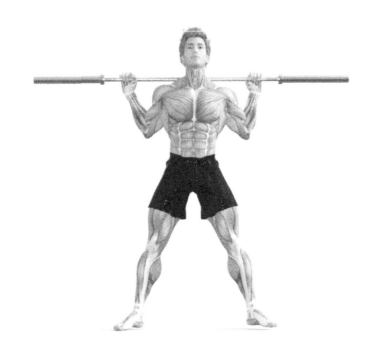

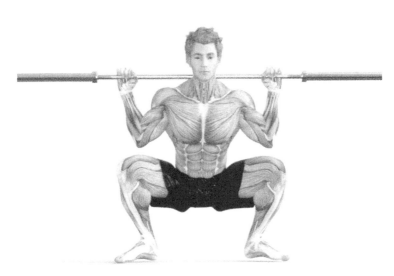

Start position

- This is a compound movement for the leg muscles
- Select a straight bar, preferably on a rack that is just below shoulder height
- Stand underneath the bar so that it rests across your trapezius and shoulder muscles
- Take the weight by straightening your legs whilst keeping your back flat and head in a neutral position
- Take a step back from the rack and set your feet so they are just outside shoulder width apart, toes turned out to align with your knees
- Keep a slight bend in your knees

Movement

- Before you start the movement, take a deep breath, engage your glutes and abdominals
- When ready, squat down by bending at the knees as if you were aiming to sit on a bench
- Your glutes will lead your upper body towards the floor
- Once your upper legs are parallel to the floor, this is the top of movement
- At this point, return to the start position by driving through your mid foot. Driving through your heels will put more emphasis on the quads
- Once you have finished your set, walk the bar back to the rack

Extra info

Sumo squats are designed to target the same muscle groups as regular squats but with a bigger emphasis on the inner legs and glutes. All principals from regular squats apply to sumo squats, but the foot positioning can be varied. If you are new to sumo squats, I would advise a narrower foot position to get used to the movement, a small increase in the stance from regular squats is a good start to enable you to develop a mind and muscle connection to the movement, some may get the hang of this quickly and it may take more time for others.

Dumbbell lunges

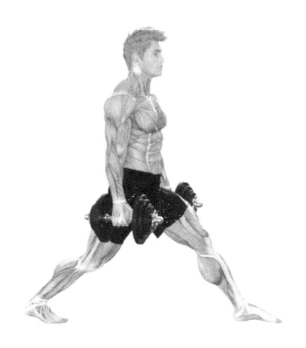

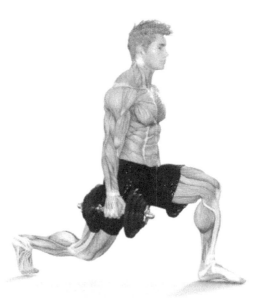

Start position

- This is a compound exercise for the leg muscles
- Select a set of dumbbells that fit with your workload, pick them up, one in each hand
- Kneel on the floors that your front leg forms a right angle from your calf to your hamstrings
- Your trailing leg should also form a right angle from the hamstrings to the calf
- The toes of your trailing leg should be in contact with the floor
- From this position, stand up with the dumbbells, arms straight but elbows slightly bent

Movement

- As you inhale, lower yourself towards the floor by bending at the knees
- Your feet should stay planted, back should stay flat and head in a neutral position
- Lower only to where the knee of the trailing leg is about to touch the floor
- Once at the top of the movement, exhale and return to the start position
- Perform a set and switch leg positions. Front leg becomes the trailing leg and vice versa

Extra info

When performing this exercise, your front knee should not move forward of your toes, this will put undue strain on the knee joints. Lunges can be performed on each leg and then the legs are switched for the second half of the set, or they can be performed as alternate lunges or walking lunges. The disadvantage here is that the setup has to be correct each time the feet are moved. More experienced trainers will have an easier time with these methods, so for new trainers to this exercise, I would advise the exercise is performed as per the description.

Dumbbell stiff leg deadlift

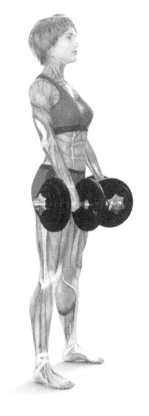

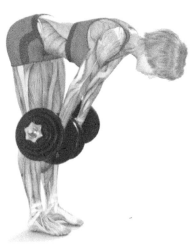

Start position

- This is an isolation exercise for the hamstrings and glutes
- Select a set of dumbbells that fit with your workload, taking an overhand grip with hands shoulder width apart
- Arms should be fully extended with a slight bend in the elbows and the dumbbells should hang close to the body, across the front of the quads
- Stand with your feet about hip width apart with your toes pointing forward
- Ensure that your back is flat and head is in a neutral position
- Keep a slight bend in the knees throughout this exercise

Movement

- Before you start the movement, engage your glutes
- As you exhale, hinge at the hips to lower your upper body towards the floor, keeping the dumbbells close to your body
- Keep your back flat and head in a neutral position
- Lower to where you feel the stretch in your hamstrings
- Once at the top of the movement, inhale as you return to the start position

Extra info

When it comes to the width of foot positioning, the same principals apply as barbell deadlift, so it's totally fine to have your feet together.

Performing deadlift with dumbbells gives us the opportunity to move each hand independently, so as we lower into the exercise, we can bring the dumbbells together so the touch, when returning to the start position, we can also reverse this and finish with the dumbbells by our sides, palms facing inwards.

This is more comfortable for some trainers, but if you decide to try this out, remember to keep the dumbbells controlled and keep them close to the body throughout the movement. A bit more focus may be required for this.

Bicep exercises

Straight bar curls

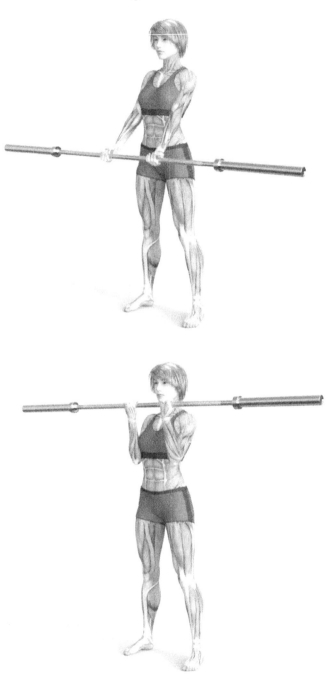

Start position

- This is a compound movement for the biceps
- Select a straight bar with a resistance that fits with your training routine
- Take an underhand grip, your hands should be in line with the front of your shoulders
- Ensure you have a flat back and head in a neutral position
- Allow the bar to hang across your upper legs, then bend your elbows slightly
- Keep a slight bend in the knees with a stance about hip width apart

Movement

- As you exhale, keeping your elbows in the start position, curl the bar upwards until your forearms are parallel with the floor
- At this point, push your elbows forward to bring the bar closer to your upper body whilst you continue to bend at the elbows until your upper arms are at about a 45-degree angle
- Once at the top of movement, inhale and return to the start position
- Elbows should never lock out at the start position, keep a slight bend in them

Extra info

I class this exercise as a compound movement as the shoulder is involved. To get the most out of this exercise, there is a slight double movement where the shoulders engage to help finish the movement, keeping tension on the biceps. It is possible to focus fully on the biceps during this movement, but I've always found more benefit from pushing the elbows forward to get a better contraction.

A point to note about bicep curls of any kind is that the wider your grip, the more focus is given to the inner head and the narrower the grip, the more focus is given to the outer head. But until a trainer notices an imbalance of the biceps, it's advised that the grip width should be "hands in line with shoulders".

EZ bar curls

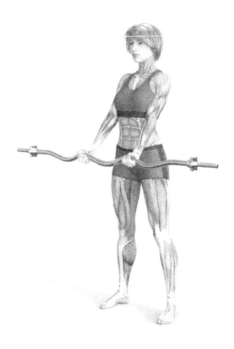

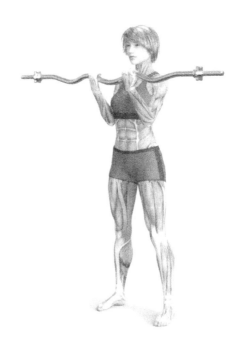

Start position

- This is a compound movement for the biceps
- Select an EZ bar with a resistance that fits with your training routine
- Take an underhand grip, your hands should be in line with the front of your shoulders
- Your grip should be on the bends of the EZ bar so your palms are facing inwards slightly
- Ensure you have a flat back and head in a neutral position
- Allow the bar to hang across your upper legs, then bend your elbows slightly
- Keep a slight bend in the knees with a stance about hip width apart

Movement

- As you exhale, keeping your elbows in the start position, curl the bar upwards until your forearms are parallel with the floor
- At this point, push your elbows forward to bring the bar closer to your upper body whilst you continue to bend at the elbows until your upper arms are at about a 45-degree angle
- Once at the top of movement, inhale and return to the start position
- Elbows should never lock out at the start position, keep a slight bend in them

Extra info

EZ bars are available with several angles to grip. Ideally, choose a bar that is not too exaggerated. The idea of this bar is to target both bicep muscles with a slight wrist rotation. Some trainers choose this exercise over a straight bar purely from a comfort point of view.

Close grip barbell curls

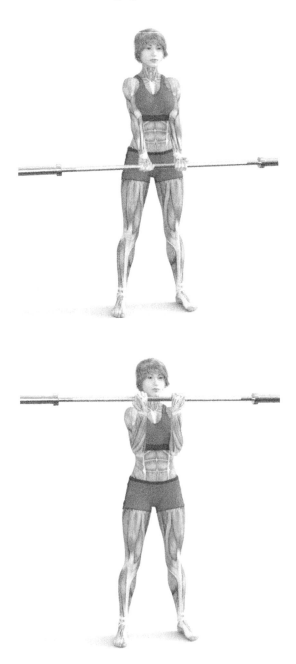

Start position

- This is a compound movement for the biceps
- Select a straight bar with a resistance that fits with your training routine
- Take an underhand grip, your hands inside your shoulders
- Ensure you have a flat back and head in a neutral position
- Allow the bar to hang across your upper legs, then bend your elbows slightly
- Keep a slight bend in the knees with a stance about hip width apart

Movement

- As you exhale, keeping your elbows in the start position, curl the bar upwards until your forearms are parallel with the floor
- At this point, push your elbows forward to bring the bar closer to your upper body whilst you continue to bend at the elbows until your upper arms are at about a 45-degree angle
- Once at the top of movement, inhale and return to the start position
- Elbows should never lock out at the start position, keep a slight bend in them

Extra info

This exercise puts a bigger focus on the outer head of the biceps. As stated previously, I would suggest that it is more relevant to trainers that have some experience in bicep curls and feel that there is a lack of development of the outer head of the biceps.

Supination curls

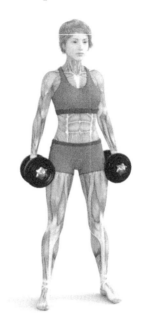

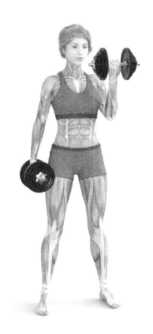

Start position

- This is a compound movement for the biceps
- Select a set of dumbbells that fit with your training routine
- Pick up the dumbbells and hold them by your sides. Your elbows should be slightly bent
- Palms should face inwards
- Ensure you have a flat back and head in a neutral position
- Knees should be slightly bent and feet shoulder width apart

Movement

- As you exhale, rotate your wrist whilst bending one arm at the elbow until your forearm is parallel to the ground
- At this point, push your elbow forward to continue the curl
- Once your upper arm is at a 45-degree angle to the floor, return to the start position as you inhale
- Repeat on the opposite arm and continue this pattern until you have completed your set

Extra info

The rotation of your wrist should be an incremental movement through the exercise. The more your elbow bends, the more your wrist rotates; you should finish rotation at the top of movement so that the dumbbell bar ends, so it's parallel to the ground. This incremental rotation movement is reversed when returning to the start position.

This exercise can be performed as single arm curls or the curls can be performed with both arms simultaneously. If you are performing the single arm version, it's easier to fall into the trap of using momentum to lift the other by leaning to the side. To guard against this, ensure that you are static before starting the movement on the opposite arm.

Dumbbell concentration curls

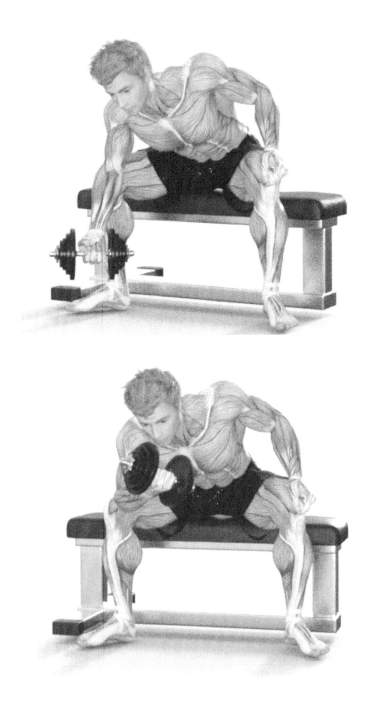

Start position

- This is an isolation movement for the biceps
- Select a dumbbell that fits with your training routine
- Sit long ways on a flat bench with your feet flat on the floor and outside your shoulders
- Place the dumbbell on the inside of your right foot
- Hinge at the hips with your working arm out in front of you until your elbow rests on the inside of your knee
- Rest your other hand on your other knee for support
- Pick up the dumbbell with your right hand and straighten your arm until you have a slight bend in the elbow
- Ensure you have a flat back and head in a neutral position

Movement

- As you exhale, curl the dumbbell up towards your upper body by bending your elbow
- Your upper arm should not move as it is kept in place with the elbow pressed into the inside of the knee
- Your back should remain flat and head in a neutral position
- Once you reach maximum contraction with in your bicep, as you inhale, return to the start position
- Once you have completed a set on one arm, mirror the start position and perform the set on the opposite arm

Extra info

This is an isolation exercise, as there is no shoulder rotation. Once this movement is perfected, the reps should feel fairly intense. Dumbbell concentration curls can be used as a pre exhaust set before doing other barbell exercises, it can also be done as a finisher for extra workout intensity. I would recommend this exercise for goals such as bodybuilding or other types of training that have an emphasis on aesthetics.

Hammer curls

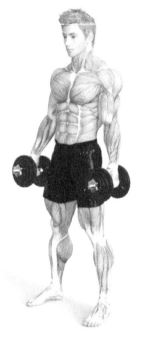

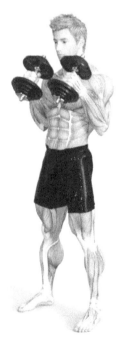

Start position

- An Isolation exercise for the biceps
- Select a set of dumbbells that fit with your training routine
- Pick up the dumbbells and hold them by your sides. Your elbows should be slightly bent
- Palms should face inwards
- Ensure you have a flat back and head in a neutral position
- Knees should be slightly bent and feet shoulder width apart

Movement

- As you exhale, bend your arms at the elbow until your forearm is parallel to the ground
- Keep your elbows in and towards your sides. The only movement should be from your elbow joint
- Once your upper arm is at a 45-degree angle to the floor, return to the start position as you inhale

Extra info

Although I have categorised this as an isolation exercise, it can easily be turned into a compound movement. If the exercise description is changed slightly and the elbows are pushed forward mid-way through the movement, it becomes a compound movement. This is perfectly fine, but it's useful to understand the slight change of movement.

Dumbbell hammer curls can be done simultaneously or as an alternate arm movement as described in the supination curl description. Again, if you decided to use the single arm method, be mindful not to use momentum to complete the reps.

Shoulder exercises

Barbell shoulder press

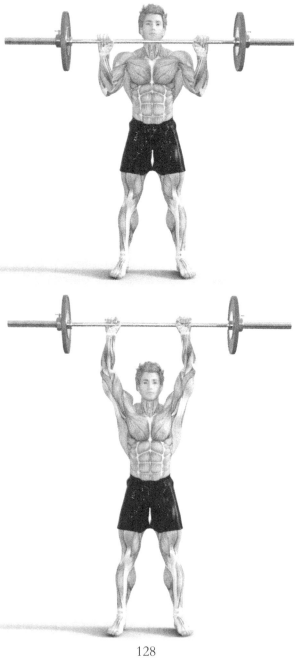

Start position

- A compound exercise for the shoulder muscles
- Select a barbell that fits with your training goals. Ideally, the barbell should be racked at about shoulder height
- With your feet about shoulder width apart, pick up the bar, taking a grip so your hands are just outside shoulder width
- The bar should be in line with your chin, back should be flat and head in the neutral position

Movement

- As you exhale, push the bar above your head until you reach a point where your arms are about to lock out
- Once you have reached the top of movement, return the bar to the start position as you inhale
- The bar should not travel lower than your chin
- Keep your back flat throughout the movement

Extra info

Barbell shoulder press is a great exercise for progression in shoulder strength and stability as it uses all three heads of the shoulders and brings in the trap muscles.

With grip width, some trainers have a narrower grip. This is ok, but a narrow grip or wider grip can cause a weaker movement. The best way to gauge your grip width is by bringing your arms up to your sides so your lower arms are parallel with the floor and directly out to your sides and forming a right angle with your lower arms. When in this position, the point at which your hands are positioned should be your grip width.

Barbell front raises

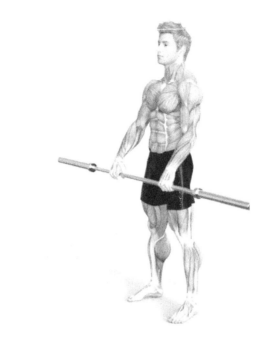

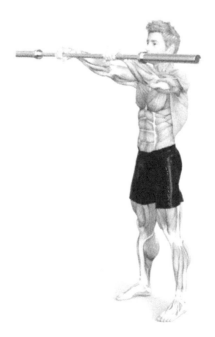

Start position

- This is an isolation exercise for the front shoulder muscles
- Select a barbell that fits with your training goals, take an overhand grip of the bar so your hands are about shoulder width apart
- Keep your back flat, head in a neutral position and keep your knees slightly bent
- Have a slight bend in your elbows and have the bar just in front of your upper legs

Movement

- As you exhale, raise the bar in front of you until it reaches about chin height
- Once at the top of movement, return the bar to the start position whilst inhaling
- Keep your elbows slightly bent and locked throughout the movement and don't swing the bar

Extra info

When raising the bar on this exercise, make sure you get to at least chin height or just above shoulder height. There is no need to raise the bar higher than this, as it can dilute the movement by taking the tension off the working muscle.

Dumbbell lateral raises

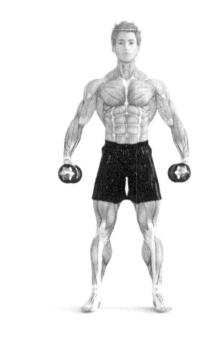

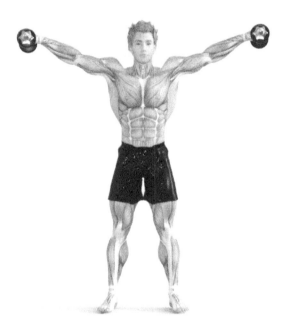

Start position

- This is an isolation exercise for the lateral shoulder muscles
- Select a set of dumbbells that fit with your training goals
- Stand with your feet hip width apart, back flat and head in a neutral position
- Hold the dumbbells by your sides with your elbows slightly bent

Movement

- As you exhale, raise the dumbbells up and out to your sides until they are just above shoulder height, or in line with your chin
- Keep your elbows slightly bent and locked throughout the movement
- Once at the top of movement, as you inhale, return to the start position

Extra info

It's common on this type of exercise to be tempted to use momentum to "swing" the dumbbells up. If you find you need to do this to complete the planned reps, the dumbbells may be too heavy, so try a lighter set. It's also common to relax between reps and lose the slight bend in the elbows whilst also losing the tension on the shoulder muscle, and we don't want this. So, it's something extra to think about during this type of exercise.

Dumbbell front raises

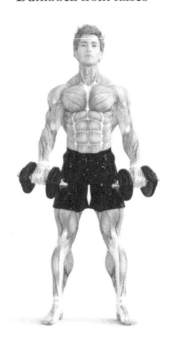

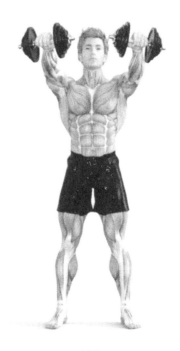

Start position

- This is an isolation exercise for the front shoulder muscles
- Select a set of dumbbells that fit with your training goals
- Keep your back flat, head in a neutral position and keep your knees slightly bent
- Have a slight bend in your elbows and have the dumbbells just in front of your upper legs

Movement

- As you exhale, raise the dumbbells in front of you until they reach about chin height or just above your shoulders
- Once at the top of movement, return the dumbbells to the start position ass you inhale
- Keep your elbows slightly bent and locked throughout the movement and don't swing the dumbbells

Extra info

When performing this exercise, some trainers have the dumbbells slightly angled or even set so the palms are facing towards the body, but in my experience, it is more beneficial to the target muscle group if the palms are parallel to the ground at the top of the movement.

Dumbbell rear delt raises

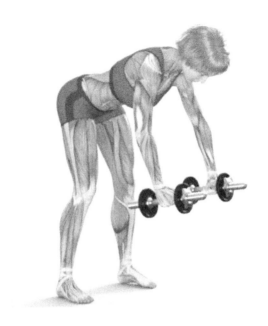

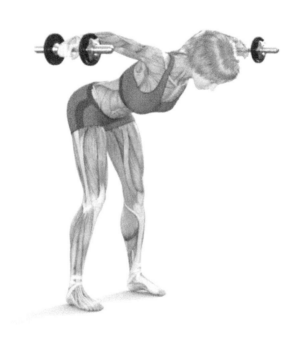

Start position

- This is an isolation exercise for the rear delts
- Pick up a set of dumbbells that fit with your goals and hold them in a hammer style, palms in
- Bend your elbows slightly, feet about shoulder width apart and hinge at the hips so your upper body is above parallel to the ground
- Back should be flat and head in a neutral position
- The dumbbells should hang in front of you

Movement

- As you exhale, raise the dumbbells upwards until they are in line or slightly above your shoulders
- Keep your back flat and head as per the start position. Your elbows should also remain in a slightly bent position
- Once at the top of movement, return to the start position as you inhale

Extra info

This can be a tricky exercise to perform correctly. I would advise doing this in front of a mirror and glancing up to check your start position and top of movement. As you are looking down throughout this movement, it can be hard to estimate the correct positions. Once you are used to how this movement feels, it will be easier to perform without a mirror.

It's common for this exercise to bend the elbows during the movement. This can dilute the workload to the rear deltoids, creating more of a row movement.

Another point to note about this is the amount of hip hinge needed, some trainers prefer to have a small, forward hip hinge, play around with this position to see what suites you, but always remember that this exercise is to target the rear deltoids, too little hip hinge can dilute the workload to the rear dealt and pull from the lateral deltoid.

Tricep exercises

Straight bar skull crushers

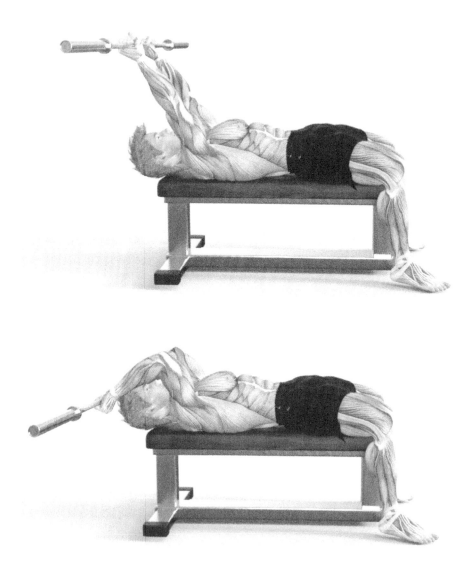

Start position

- An isolation exercise for the triceps
- Select a straight bar that fits with your training goals and a flat bench
- Lay on the bench so your feet are flat on the floor
- Grip the bar so your hands are about shoulder width apart
- Hold the bar out in front of you so it's above your mid-chest, have a slight bend in your elbows
- From this position, bring the bar to position it over your head slightly. Your arms should be at about a 45-degree angle from your body

Movement

- As you exhale, keep your upper arm in the start position but bend your elbows so the bar lowers towards your head
- The bar should not touch your head, the top of movement should be about an inch away
- Once at the top of movement, as you inhale, return to the start position

Extra info

The most common mistake on this exercise is not getting the start position right. Moving your upper arms to a 45-degree angle makes a lot of difference. From this position, the triceps are worked to maximum contraction and extension. The only joint moving in this exercise is the elbow joint.

For some trainers, it can be a bit disorientating to train in this position, and the fear of falling off the bench or feeling unstable can put trainers off. If you have these feelings, try widening your foot stance for better stability.

EZ bar scull crushers

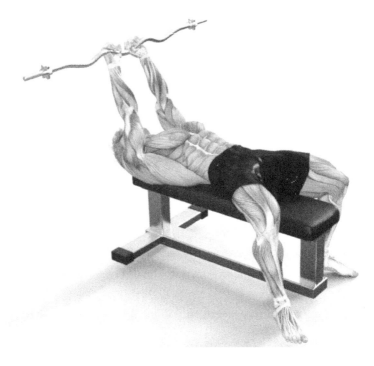

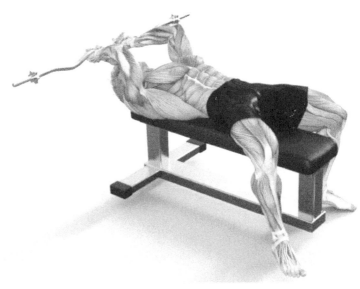

Start position

- An isolation exercise for the triceps
- Select an EZ bar that fits with your training goals and a flat bench
- Lay on the bench so your feet are flat on the floor
- Grip the bar so your hands fit into either the wider arcs or the narrower arcs on the bar
- Hold the bar out in front of you so it's above your mid-chest, have a slight bend in your elbows
- From this position, bring the bar to position it over your head slightly. Your arms should be at about a 45-degree angle from your body

Movement

- As you exhale, keep your upper arm in the start position but bend your elbows so the bar lowers towards your head
- The bar should not touch your head, the top of movement should be about an inch away
- Once at the top of movement, as you inhale, return to the start position

Extra info

Should you use a wide grip or narrow grip? Ultimately, the hand space on this exercise should be determined by comfort. With that said, a wider grip will train all three of the triceps heads more evenly, but this can be uncomfortable for some trainers. The ideal hand spacing should be about shoulder width apart or slightly wider and many EZ bars are set up for this.

If you feel discomfort in your shoulders when performing this exercise, try making your grip a bit narrower. Maybe you have to play around with your hand spacing to find what works for you.

Overhead tricep extensions (seated)

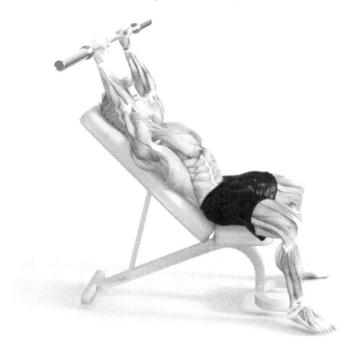

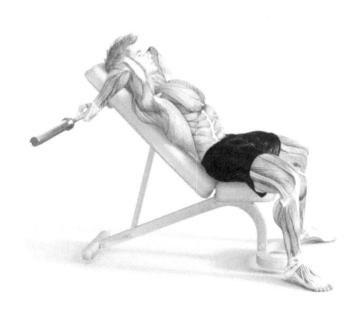

Start position

- This is an isolation exercise for the triceps
- Set an incline bench up with about a 45-degree angle
- Select a barbell and grip it with hands spaced about shoulder width apart
- Sit on the bench, keeping your back flat, head in a neutral position and feet flat on the floor
- Raise the bar directly above your head with straight arms but keep a slight bend in the elbows
- From this position, raise your arms a little more so that your triceps extend

Movement

- As you inhale, lower the bar behind your head until you feel the stretch on your triceps
- Your upper arms should stay in the start position
- Your elbows should not have an excessive flare
- Once at the top of the movement, exhale as you return to the start position

Extra info

Some trainers find this type of tricep exercise less disorientating than skull crusher movements and will choose this over them. Remember to keep your feet flat on the floor and back flat against the bench. This exercise requires a bit more concentration than skull crushers as it can place more strain on the rotator cuff when compared to skull crushers, so take extra care with this one.

Tricep extensions (hand and knee on bench)

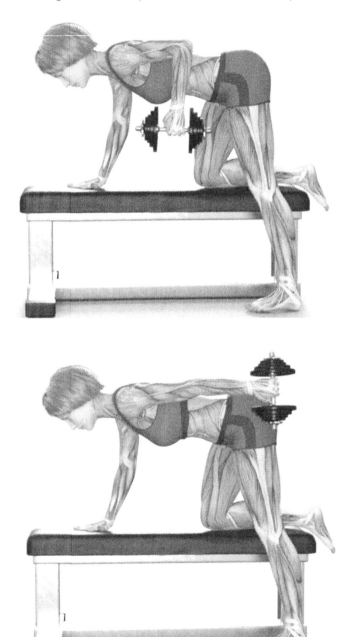

Start position

- An isolation exercise for the triceps
- Select a dumbbell that fits with your training goals and a flat bench
- Place one knee and the palm of the same side on the bench. Your other foot should be flat on the floor
- Keep your back flat and head in a neutral position
- Pick up the dumbbell with your free hand and row it towards your torso
- Your upper arm should be just above parallel to the floor

Movement

- As you exhale, raise your lower arm by bending at the elbow so the dumbbell up and past your hip
- Your upper arm should stay fixed in the start position
- Once at the top of movement, as you inhale, lower the dumbbell to the start position
- Once you have completed a set, switch arms and repeat on the other side

Extra info

I would advise that beginners try other tricep exercises before jumping into this, as it requires a bit more coordination than skull crushers, for instance. I also believe that to get the most out of this exercise, a basic foundation of tricep strength and "mind muscle connection" is needed. With this said, if you are a beginner, try it out and find that it's effective, go for it!

Another tip for this exercise is to perform it side on to a mirror so you can glance up and check your positioning. It's easy to flare your arms out or lower your upper arm during the set, which will dilute the effectiveness of the exercise.

Abs And Core

Although this book is focused on barbells and dumbbells and abdominals are limited to pretty much limited to stabiliser muscles, it's always good to keep them involved and target them as they were any other muscle group. I've decided to add the abdominal exercises from my previous book "Body weight training and calisthenics" for you to refer to, not just as shameless plug for this guide, it should be useful too. One thing I would preface this with is that when training with barbells and dumbbells, you should always put abdominal exercises at the end of your workout.

This is because every other exercise will need to call upon the abs for support. If the abs are fatigued when they are needed as stabilisers muscles, this can affect your exercise form, and even cause injury.

Excerpt from "bodyweight training & Calisthenics" begins

I have always found it useful to look at the abs in two parts, the upper section and the lower section, and for a solid all over abs workout, you should target both areas. One rule that is super helpful in figuring out which abs exercises target which area is:

If your legs are being drawn up towards your chests, this is a lower abs exercise.

If your head and chest are being drawn towards your legs, it's an upper abs exercise.

Of course, either type of ab exercise will have an engagement of both the upper and lower, but if you want to target either part of the abs individually, you can follow this rule.

An example of an upper ab exercise is the well-known "Crunch" or "Sit up" and an example of a lower ab exercise is the "knee raise".

This is a guide to effective resistance training with a focus on full body workouts. So I have included some abdominal and lower back exercises.

If you are training with a resistance routine, and you are performing the exercises with good form, you will engage your abdominal muscles through every rep of every set for all the exercises choices. This promotes core strength and good posture.

Exercises that directly target the abdominals can be used to further strengthen these muscles. When targeting the abs with specific exercises, they should always be among the last exercises in your training session. This is because they are used as support and stabilisation for all other exercises and you don't want them to be fatigued early in your training session.

The same goes for lower back movements. Lower back muscles can be strengthened and conditioned with specific exercises. Lower back pain is a very common problem and, in most cases, strong lower back muscles and good lower back mobility can prevent this. So consider adding a lower back exercise or two to the end of your routine.

Upper abs

1st progression – Seated crunch

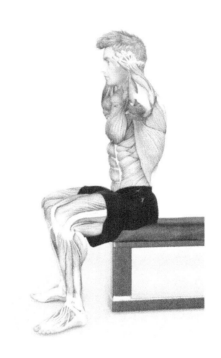

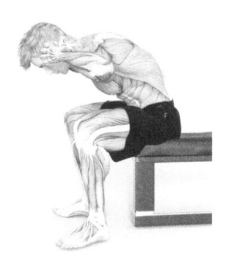

Start position

- You will need a bench or sturdy chair
- Sit on the bench so that your back is flat, abs are engaged, your head is in the neutral position, your feet are flat on the floor and they are just past shoulder width apart
- Bring your arms up and place your fingers on your temples

Movement

- As you exhale, hinge at your hips and round your back to "crunch" your abdominal muscles
- Keep your feet flat on the floor, head in the neutral position and shoulders remaining back and down
- Once at the top of the movement, inhale and return to the start position

Extra info

Breathing correctly in every exercise is important, but with abdominal exercises in particular, the correct breathing pattern will help the movement significantly. Exhaling while performing the crunch will actually start the exercise for you. Remember not to round your shoulders and to keep your feet planted on the floor.

2nd progression – Crunches, wrists to knees

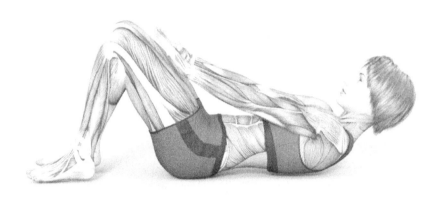

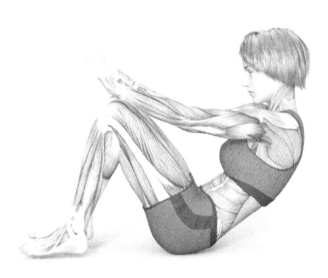

Start position

- Lay flat on the floor so your back, the back of your head and backs of your legs make full contact
- Bring your knees up towards your chest by putting both feet flat on the floor. Keep your knees together. Your heels should be close to your glutes
- Lift your head and shoulders off the floor by engaging your abdominals
- Straighten your arms so that your palms are flat against the front of your quads
- With your abdominals engaged, tilt your hips slightly to push your lower back into the floor

Movement

- As you exhale, arch your back to "crunch" your abdominal muscles
- Keep your arms straight, but slide your palms down your quads until your wrists are in contact with your knees
- Once at the top of movement, inhale and return to the start, position under control

Extra info

One of the more common mistakes with abdominal exercises is not observing the "hip tilt". A good set of crunches will maintain lower back contact with the floor. This will not only protect the lower back, but it will engage deep core muscles and offer a much more efficient abdominal workout.

When returning to the start position between reps, it may be tempting to put your head and shoulders back on the floor, but this should be avoided. If the start position is relaxed, the tension will be lost from the abdominal muscles, causing a dilution of the set.

The "wrist to knees" part of this exercise is predominantly a gauge for range of movement. It's a relatively small movement, but this depth gauge can help beginner trainers with the familiarisation of abdominal engagement and prep for future progressions.

3rd progression – Crunches, fingers on temples

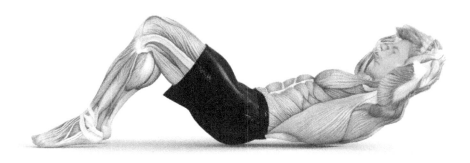

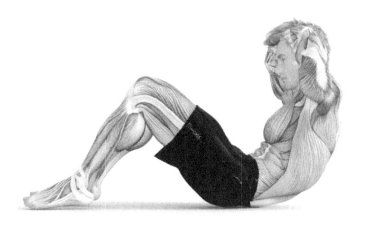

Start position

- Lay flat on the floor so your back, the back of your head and backs of your legs make full contact
- Bring your knees up towards your chest by putting both feet flat on the floor
- Lift your head and shoulders off the floor by engaging your abdominals
- Bring your arms elbows up so that your fingers are resting on your temples
- With your abdominals engaged, tilt your hips slightly to push your lower back into the floor

Movement

- As you exhale, arch your back to "crunch" your abdominal muscles
- Keep your feet firmly planted on the floor and lower back in contact with the floor
- Keep your head in the neutral position and fingers on your temples
- Once at the top of movement, inhale and return to the start, position under control

Extra info

With this exercise as a progression from the previous, we have no "depth gauge" so you should aim for maximum contraction of your abdominal muscles whilst being conscious of your lower back in contact with the floor. This may take some practice to become comfortable with, but it is an important part of abdominal and core development.

When working towards maximum range of movement, it is common to tuck the chin or bring the elbows towards the midline of the body. This will cause loss of form and alignment and dilute the workload. So be aware of this too.

4th progression – Crunches on exercise ball

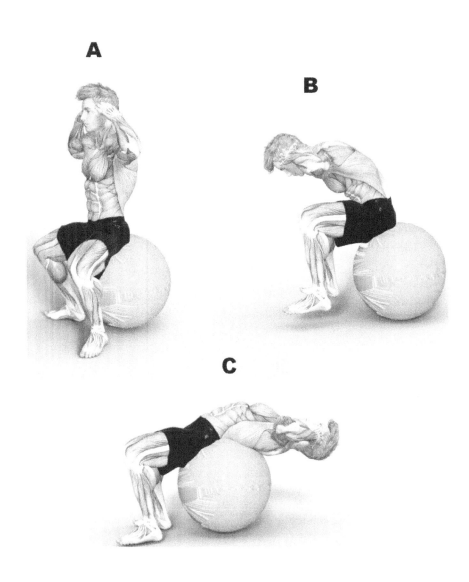

Start position "A"

- You will need an exercise ball
- Sit on the exercise ball so that your back is flat, abs are engaged, your head is in the neutral position, your feet are flat on the floor and they are just past shoulder width apart
- Bring your arms up and place your fingers on your temples

Movement "B"

- As you inhale, hinge at the hips to lean backwards over the ball
- Whilst leaning backwards, if needed, walk your feet forward, allowing the ball to roll up your back
- Once the ball is resting in the small of your back, plant your feet and lean back further to hyperextend your back slightly
- You should feel the stretch on your abdominals

Movement "C"

- As you exhale, arch your back to "crunch" your abdominal muscles.
- Keep your feet firmly planted on the floor.
- Keep your head in the neutral position and fingers on your temples.
- Once at the top of movement, inhale and return to the start, position under control.

Extra info

This exercise does require a specific piece of exercise kit, but it is excellent to use as a full range of motion movement.

If you decide to add this to your exercise routine and have trouble balancing on the ball, widening your feet should help with this. If you want to make this more challenging, bring your feet closer together.

5th progression – Crunches feet raised

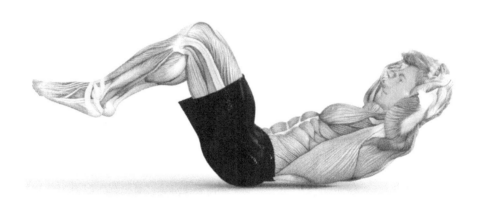

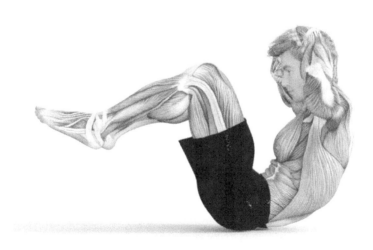

Start position

- Lay flat on the floor and bring your knees up towards your chest, bringing your feet into an elevated position
- Lift your head and shoulders off the floor by engaging your abdominals
- Bring your arms elbows up so that your fingers are resting on your temples
- With your abdominals engaged, tilt your hips slightly to push your lower back into the floor

Movement

- As you exhale, arch your back to "crunch" your abdominal muscles
- Keep your feet elevated and lower back in contact with the floor
- Keep your head in the neutral position and fingers on your temples
- Once at the top of movement, inhale and return to the start, position under control

Extra info

This can be a challenging upgrade for many people. If you are finding the progression too tough, try holding the start position and use it as an isometric exercise. Concentrate on the hip tilt that pushes your lower back into the floor whilst making sure that your feet are stable in the elevated position.

Once you get comfortable with this, try smaller crunch movements rather than a full crunch and work towards range of movement progression in future workouts.

6th progression – V Sit

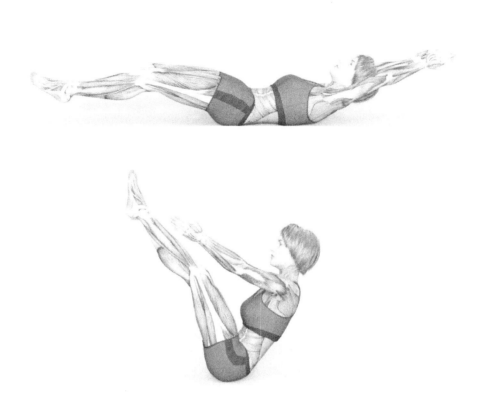

Start position

- Lay flat on the floor keeping your legs straight and together, but ensure to maintain a small bend in the knees
- Tilt your hips slightly to push your lower back into the floor
- Engage your abdominals and glutes and lift your heels off the floor about an inch
- Lift your head and shoulders off the floor while keeping your abdominals engaged
- Bring your arms up so that they are straight with a slight bend in the elbows above your head

Movement

- As you exhale, roll your upper body off the floor whilst simultaneously raising your legs
- Keep your arms straight with a slight bend at the elbows forward, towards your feet
- Your leg lock position should also be maintained and head in the neutral position
- Ensure that your abdominals and glutes are engaged throughout the movement
- Once you have formed a "V" shape with your body and you are balancing on your glutes, this is the top of movement. Inhale and return to the start position under control

Extra info

This is an advanced movement and should only be attempted by trainers that have a strong core. A common mistake with this exercise is to use momentum to perform the movement; this significantly reduces the intended training effect. The exercise should be performed under control with strict form.

Also, it is important to keep your shoulder alignment with this exercise. It can be tempting to "reach" with your arms towards your feet, causing rounding of the shoulders. The last thing to note with this exercise is that when returning to the start position, you should always maintain.

If you become competent at this exercise and would like a further challenge, when at the top of the movement, try pausing for a second or two before returning to the start position.

Lower abs

1st progression – Lying knee raise, single leg

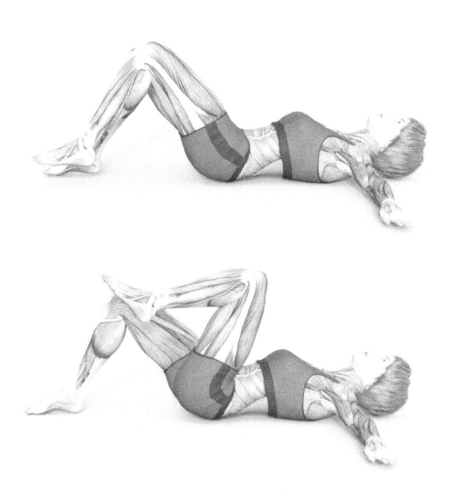

Start position

- Lay flat on the floor, have your legs bent so your feet are flat to the floor and about hip width apart
- Tilt your hips slightly to push your lower back into the floor
- Engage your abdominals and glutes and lift one foot about an inch off the floor. This will be the "moving leg
- Place your arms out to your sides, palms down and flat to the floor for stability
- Ensure that your head and back are in contact with the floor throughout the movement

Movement

- As you exhale, raise your "moving leg" up towards your chest until your lower leg is parallel with the floor
- Your knees should remain at the same angel as the starting position
- The position of your head, back and arms should be maintained throughout the movement
- Once you are at the top of the movement, inhale and return to the start position
- When you have completed the planned reps for this exercise, repeat for the other leg

Extra info

When returning to the start position with this exercise, you should not return the foot of the "moving leg" back to the floor, always maintain a small gap.

Be conscious of lower back position and keep awareness of hip alignment. Once fatigue starts to kick in, it may be tempting for one side of your lower back or glutes to lift off the floor. If you feel this happening, fix it immediately, or finish the exercise if it is indeed due to fatigue.

2nd progression – Double knee raise

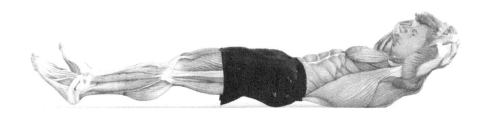

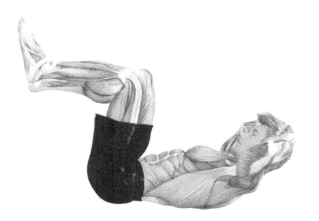

Start position

- Lay flat on the floor, keeping your legs straight and feet about hip width apart
- Tilt your hips slightly to push your lower back into the floor
- Engage your abdominals and glutes and lift both feet about an inch off the floor
- Bring your head and shoulders off the floor to engage your abdominals
- Raise your arms and hands to place your fingers on your temples

Movement

- As you exhale, raise both legs up towards your chest whilst also bending your knees, until your lower legs are parallel with the floor
- The position of your head, back and arms should be maintained throughout the movement
- Once you are at the top of the movement, inhale and return to the start position

Extra info

If you find this is too much of a progression, you can change the tart position slightly by keeping your head and back flat to the floor and placing your arms out to your sides, palms down and flat to the floor for stability. This is the same upper body starting position as the previous progression.

It's also important for this exercise to be aware of using momentum to perform the movement. It can be tempting to "bounce" or "jolt" your legs to kick-start the movement. We want to avoid this, as it can dilute the workload from our target muscle groups.

3rd progression – Leg raise

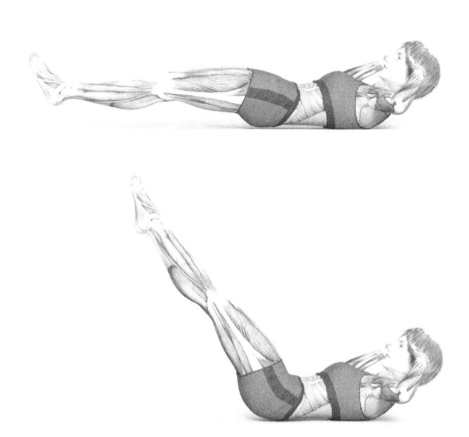

Start position

- Lay flat on the floor, keeping your legs straight and close together
- Tilt your hips slightly to push your lower back into the floor
- Engage your abdominals and glutes and lift both feet about an inch off the floor
- Bring your head and shoulders off the floor to engage your abdominals
- Raise your arms and hands to place your fingers on your temples

Movement

- As you exhale, raise both legs up towards your chest, keeping them straight. You should stop just before your legs are vertical
- The position of your head, back and arms should be maintained throughout the movement
- Once you are at the top of the movement, inhale and return to the start position

Extra info

With this progression, there will be a bigger temptation to use momentum to perform the movement than the previous one, so, again, be aware. Also, you can also place your arms and head on the floor for stability if you find this to be too much of a progression from the previous exercise. If you choose this option, be aware that it will be much easier to lose your lower back stability by pulling it away from the floor.

4th progression Seated knee raise

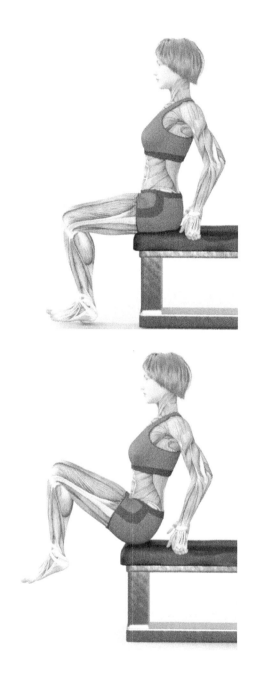

Start position

- You will need a bench, strong chair or equivalent
- Sit on the bench so that your back is flat, abs are engaged, your head is in the neutral position
- Your legs and feet should be together and lifted off the floor slightly
- Grip the sides of the bench with your palms facing in

Movement

- As you exhale, lift your knees towards your chest
- Ensure that you maintain a flat back and natural head position
- Once your upper legs reach a 45-degree angle, this is the top of the movement
- Inhale and return to the starting position

Extra info

Again, be aware of using momentum, but with this exercise, there may be temptation to arch your back and bring your shoulders forward to complete the movement. Always keep your back flat, abs and glutes engaged and use your grip on the bench for stability if this happens.

Remember when returning to the start position to keep your feet about an inch away from the floor. This will keep tension in the abdominals and give a more efficient workout.

5th progression Hanging Knee raise

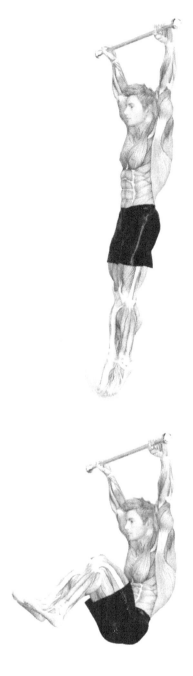

Start position

- You will need a pull-up bar or an equivalent piece of kit
- Your hands should grip the bar so that they are just past the line of your outer shoulders
- Have your feet and knees together, legs straight, but maintain a slight bend in the knees
- Engage your core and glutes to bring your legs forward slightly
- Engage your traps and lats by pulling your shoulders slightly back and down, whilst also slightly pulling your elbows down. This will create a slight bend in the elbows
- Keep your head facing forward or looking up slightly

Movement

- As you exhale, bend your knees slightly to tuck your lower legs. Bring your legs up towards your chest until your quads form a 45-degree angle with your upper body
- Ensure that you hinge at the hips to fully engage the lower abdominals
- Once at the top of movement, inhale and return to the start, position under control

Extra info

As you tuck your lower legs, it may be tempting to use the momentum to complete the movement. To avoid this, you may want to tuck your legs before you start the movement. But tucking your lower legs as you perform the movement will help towards the next progression. The longer that your legs stay straight, the more that this exercise looks like the next progression. This is an exercise that helps to practise as technique plays a part, so have a practice, but remember the fundamentals and what the exercise is designed to do.

6th progression Hanging leg raise

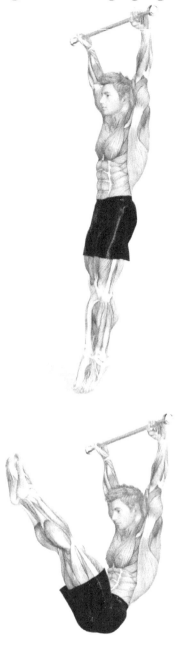

Start position

- You will need a pull-up bar or an equivalent piece of kit
- Your hands should grip the bar so that they are just past the line of your outer shoulders
- Have your feet and knees together, legs straight, but maintain a slight bend in the knees
- Engage your core and glutes to bring your legs forward slightly
- Engage your traps and lats by pulling your shoulders slightly back and down, whilst also slightly pulling your elbows down. This will create a slight bend in the elbows
- Keep your head facing forward or looking up slightly

Movement

- As you exhale, bring your legs up towards your chest until they form a 45-degree angle with your upper body
- Maintain the start position for your lower legs and upper body
- Ensure that you hinge at the hips to fully engage the lower abdominals
- Once at the top of movement, inhale and return to the start, position under control

Extra info

If you find that this is too much of a progression, you can complete the exercise with bent legs. If you choose to do this, bend your legs at the knee to tuck your lower legs at the start of the movement. Maintain this leg position throughout the movement.

To ensure that you get the most value from this exercise, concentrate on control, both on the leg elevation and when returning to the start position.

When reaching the top of movement, ensure that you are aiming for maximum contraction. Your hips should tilt forward and your lower back should be rounded. This is the benchmark.

Excerpt from "bodyweight training & Calisthenics" ends

Thank you! If you found this useful I'd like to help further…

First off, I would like to thank you for your purchase. It really means a lot that you spent your time on this guide. I am a self-published author with a passion for training and helping people get to where they want to be with fitness and by reading; you are supporting me and fuelling my passion.

This guide should give you a brilliant start in the world of bodyweight training and the planning that goes with it. But this is not my first fitness book! I've been writing and self-publishing for several years. I've written books on fitness motivation, planning, bodybuilding, home workouts and long distance running. These guides are based on my experience and formal education.

I've been a long distance endurance runner, a competing bodybuilder, and I have worked with personal training clients to change their lives through fitness, so I have a lot to share.

If you found this short guide useful and would like to read more about body transformations, fitness motivation, home workouts or more about resistance training and would like a clear path to follow, I have plenty more for you to look at including workbooks and journals for you to plan and track!

Most of my books are available in eBook and paperback format, and some are also available as audio titles narrated by an exceptional voice actor called Matt Addis.

Each fitness book is written as a standalone guide but also has its place as part of a series. So if you are a total beginner and want to become a bodybuilder or marathon runner as an end goal, I have you covered! Jump in at the start of the series with *"Fitness & Exercise Motivation"* and follow the steps, I'll be at the starting blocks with you and we will cross the finish line together!

If you would like to learn more about this series and my other books, you can do so by visiting my author page. Visit Amazon and search "James Atkinson", you will see my ugly mug, click it, and you should be taken to my page ☺

As we all know, diet plays a big part in health and fitness, and the two subjects fit hand in hand. So I would like to offer you a free download of seven healthy recipes that I created and use regularly myself. You can copy the recipes exactly, add your own twist to them, or simply take inspiration from them.

If you would like to grab this, you can do so by following the link below.

jimshealthandmuscle.com/healthy-recipes-sign-up

Remember The Podcast!

Trying to create an online business is tough, especially in the fitness niche! There is a lot of noise, "fairy-tale" fitness supplements, big personalities, and celebrities with huge online followings pushing their fitness ideas that often drown out the information that will actually make the difference.

In an attempt to widen my online reach, I created a podcast that is designed for the beginner who really wants to get results from their efforts. I set out to create bite sized podcast episodes of around twenty minutes that gave honest, actionable advice to the listener. This is still in its early stages, but I have to say that I've absolutely loved doing these podcast episodes and it is something that I plan to get stuck into more in the future.

If you are interested in fitness podcasts, you can find mine at Audiofittest.com

Or search Audiofittest wherever you get your podcasts from.

AudioFitTest.com

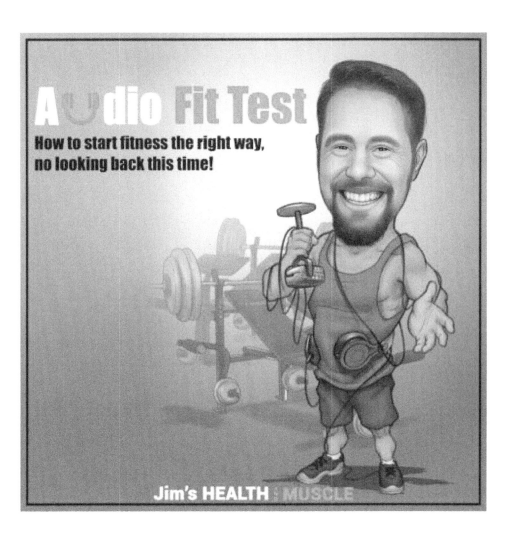

It would be great to have you along! If you do stop by, I would also really appreciate "Likes", "follows" and reviews. These things really help! The same goes for Amazon reviews for the books. If you have chance and you found the book useful, it would mean the world to me if you left a star rating and a short review.

Thanks again for your support and I wish you all the best with your training. Remember, I am always happy to help where I can, so if you have any questions, just give me a shout!

All the best,

Jim

Also by James Atkinson

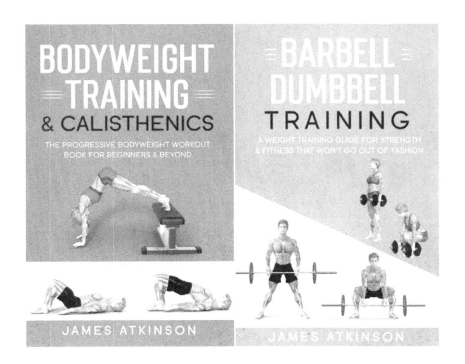

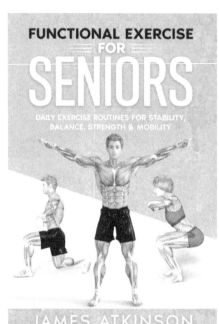

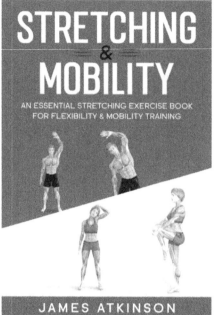

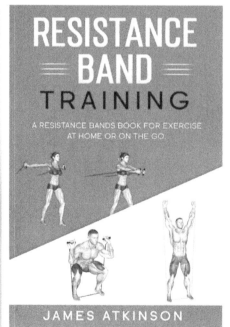

Blank Program Cards

BARBELL & DUMBBELL TRAINING

FULL BODY ROUTINE

EXERCISE	SETS	REPS	RESISTANCE

WEEKS	MON	TUE	WED	THURS	FRI	SAT	SUN
1							
2							
3							
4							
5							

BARBELL & DUMBBELL TRAINING			
FULL BODY ROUTINE			
EXERCISE	SETS	REPS	RESISTANCE

WEEKS	MON	TUE	WED	THURS	FRI	SAT	SUN
1							
2							
3							
4							
5							

BARBELL & DUMBBELL TRAINING

FULL BODY ROUTINE

EXERCISE	SETS	REPS	RESISTANCE

WEEKS	MON	TUE	WED	THURS	FRI	SAT	SUN
1							
2							
3							
4							
5							

BARBELL & DUMBBELL TRAINING			

FULL BODY ROUTINE			

EXERCISE	SETS	REPS	RESISTANCE

WEEKS	MON	TUE	WED	THURS	FRI	SAT	SUN
1							
2							
3							
4							
5							

BARBELL & DUMBBELL TRAINING

BODYBUILDING 2 DAY SPLIT TRAINING 2 DAY SPLIT

EXERCISE	SETS	REPS	RESISTANCE

WORKOUT "A"

WORKOUT "B"

WEEKS	MON	TUE	WED	THURS	FRI	SAT	SUN
1							
2							
3							
4							
5							

BARBELL & DUMBBELL TRAINING

BODYBUILDING 2 DAY SPLIT TRAINING 2 DAY SPLIT

EXERCISE	SETS	REPS	RESISTANCE

WORKOUT "A"

WORKOUT "B"

WEEKS	MON	TUE	WED	THURS	FRI	SAT	SUN
1							
2							
3							
4							
5							

BARBELL & DUMBBELL TRAINING

BODYBUILDING 2 DAY SPLIT TRAINING 2 DAY SPLIT

EXERCISE	SETS	REPS	RESISTANCE

WORKOUT "A"

WORKOUT "B"

WEEKS	MON	TUE	WED	THURS	FRI	SAT	SUN
1							
2							
3							
4							
5							

BARBELL & DUMBBELL TRAINING

BODYBUILDING 2 DAY SPLIT TRAINING 2 DAY SPLIT

EXERCISE	SETS	REPS	RESISTANCE

WORKOUT "A"

WORKOUT "B"

WEEKS	MON	TUE	WED	THURS	FRI	SAT	SUN
1							
2							
3							
4							
5							

BARBELL & DUMBBELL TRAINING			
CIRCUIT ROUTINE			
EXERCISE	REPS	RESISTANCE	SETS

WEEKS	MON	TUE	WED	THURS	FRI	SAT	SUN
1							
2							
3							
4							
5							

BARBELL & DUMBBELL TRAINING			
CIRCUIT ROUTINE			
EXERCISE	REPS	RESISTANCE	SETS

WEEKS	MON	TUE	WED	THURS	FRI	SAT	SUN
1							
2							
3							
4							
5							

BARBELL & DUMBBELL TRAINING

CIRCUIT ROUTINE

EXERCISE	REPS	RESISTANCE	SETS

WEEKS	MON	TUE	WED	THURS	FRI	SAT	SUN
1							
2							
3							
4							
5							

BARBELL & DUMBBELL TRAINING

CIRCUIT ROUTINE

EXERCISE	REPS	RESISTANCE	SETS

WEEKS	MON	TUE	WED	THURS	FRI	SAT	SUN
1							
2							
3							
4							
5							

BARBELL & DUMBBELL TRAINING

CIRCUIT ROUTINE

EXERCISE	REPS	RESISTANCE	SETS

WEEKS	MON	TUE	WED	THURS	FRI	SAT	SUN
1							
2							
3							
4							
5							

Made in the USA
Las Vegas, NV
13 July 2024